Planting Seeds

YOGA FOR KIDS
Lesson Plans for the Teacher

A Yoga and Mindfulness
for Children Series

Book 1: *Planting Seeds*

Book 2: *Peace Begins With Me*

Book 3: *Reach for the Stars*

Book 4: *We are All in this Together*

Book 5: *My Amazing Body*

Book 6: *What's Bugging You?*

Book 7: *The Elements*

Book 8: *What's the Weather?*

Planting Seeds

Growing Mindful Children
Through Yoga

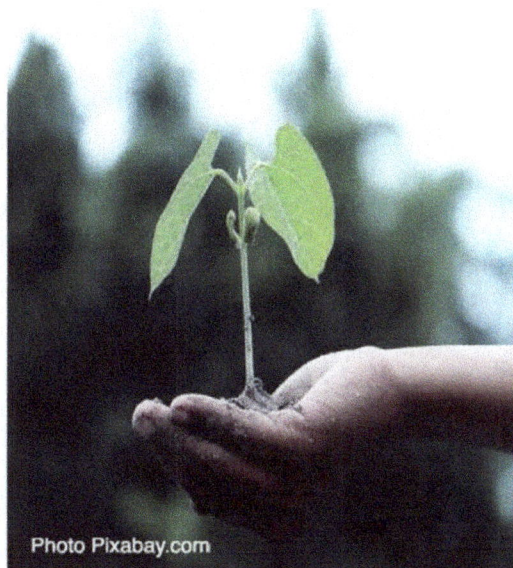

Photo Pixabay.com

Planting Seeds

Growing Mindful Children Through Yoga

FIRST EDITION

YOGA FOR KIDS
Lesson Plans for the Teacher
Book 1

Soft Cover ISBN: 979-8-9887936-0-1

**Dedicated to
Our Children**

the ones we've taught,

the ones we have yet to meet,

and the ones we raised.

Table of Contents

Border art: Pixabay.com

It is not
what is poured
into a student
that counts, but
what is planted.

~Linda Conway

Introduction

Namasté.

Yoga for children is a whole new breed of yoga! Welcome to this exciting world.

While maintaining the principles of yoga, we must tailor classes to meet the developmental needs of the age group we are working with. It would be silly to expect a group of 3- and 4-year-olds to sit in meditation for any length of time, or to breathe quietly in a pranayama (breath work) exercise. So we infuse these ideas and techniques into play.

Children learn **focus and concentration** through pose challenges and memory games. They learn **mindfulness** by listening to a bell ring or watching a glitter jar settle. They learn to **focus on their breath** by blowing bubbles and feathers. And they learn **compassion and empathy** by taking turns, playing a smile game, and looking each other in the eyes.

Schools, preschools, learning centers, parents, and teachers all recognize the value of increased focus and attention in children. We work hard to teach social skills such as team work, communication, and compassionate listening. We help children learn to self-regulate their behavior by recognizing and appropriately expressing their emotions. Yoga can be a tool to help achieve all these goals, and it works in a variety of situations: at home, in small groups, and in classrooms.

Though it is not limited to this format, this curriculum is designed as a 6-week program. Each lesson can be done as one unit in a single setting, or broken apart into several shorter sessions. Each unit lends itself to extension activities and discussions, depending on time. This is a guide to introduce yoga principles and tie them to learning. It is designed to be fun, engaging, and helpful. While it is tailored for children aged 5-12, the lessons can be modified to work in older and younger age groups.

Our hope is that yoga and its benefits become accessible to all children, and that through the introduction of important skills at a young age, we raise future generations who are caring, compassionate, confident, and empathetic.

Thank you for sharing your love of yoga with the children of the world!

Blessings,

Lenora and Janice

We welcome your feedback!
play@omtastic-yoga.com
www.omtastic-yoga.com

Follow Omtastic Yoga on Facebook
for events and lots of free ideas!

> Welcome to *"Planting Seeds"* a 6-lesson journey of movement and mindfulness with a focus on science, nature, and growth.

In this curriculum, we use the theme "Planting Seeds" to discuss two different topics:

1. How do plants grow?

    What do plants need to grow?
- Sunlight
- Water
- Air
- Earth

    How do we get more plants?
    Life cycle of plants:
- Plant seeds
- Seeds grow
- Plants produce fruit
- Seeds fall to the ground

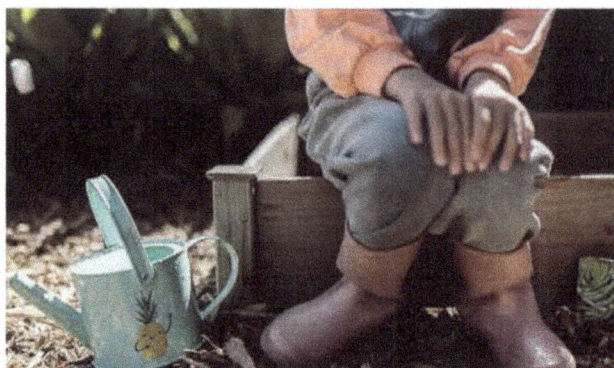

Photo: Pixabay.com

2. How do we "plant seeds" in our lives?

    What kind of seeds do we want to plant? (Principles of Yoga Tree)
- Seeds of gratitude (bringing happiness into our lives)
- Seeds of caring (care for self, others, our communities)
- Seeds of truthfulness
- Seeds of compassion (selfless-ness)
- Seeds of peace

Our Lesson Plans

Over the years, we have discovered the benefits of creating a yoga series with a theme. Returning students always have new materials and topics to work with, and students new to yoga will not feel left behind. Using themes helps connect the class to subjects from school, such as social studies, geography, and science.

You will see familiar categories in all of our lessons, such as "Focus," "Affirmation," "Breath," etc. These are consistent in almost every class we teach, although they may be presented in different orders from week to week. We have found that our students like the routine of familiar categories each week, and keeping each category brief helps keep students engaged.

Our lesson plans are guides for you to use however you like. As in yoga class, we invite you to embrace what feels right for you and your students, adapt what you feel needs modification, and disregard any activities or suggestions that are not a fit for your group.

Principles of Yoga

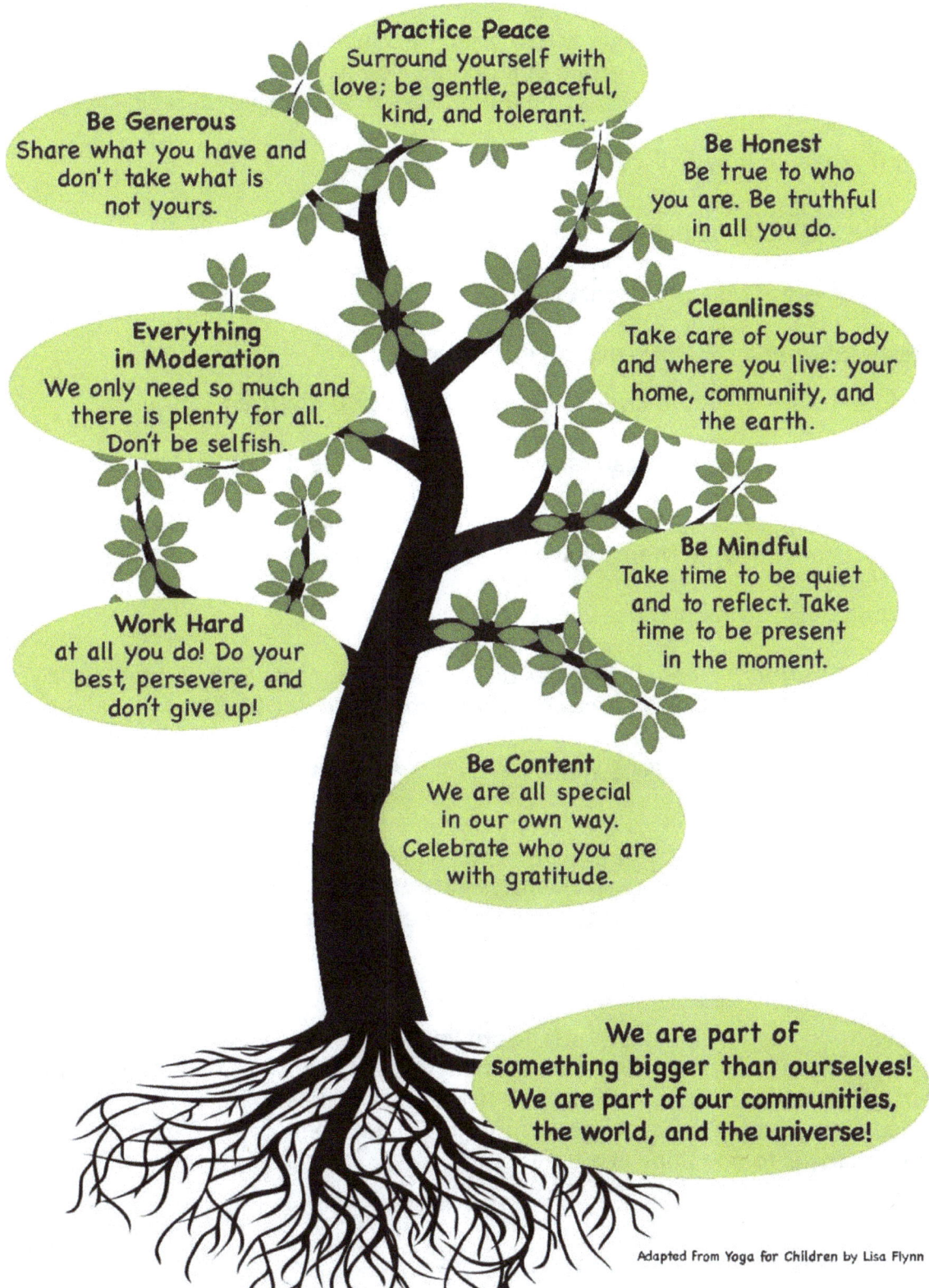

Practice Peace
Surround yourself with love; be gentle, peaceful, kind, and tolerant.

Be Generous
Share what you have and don't take what is not yours.

Be Honest
Be true to who you are. Be truthful in all you do.

Everything in Moderation
We only need so much and there is plenty for all. Don't be selfish.

Cleanliness
Take care of your body and where you live: your home, community, and the earth.

Be Mindful
Take time to be quiet and to reflect. Take time to be present in the moment.

Work Hard
at all you do! Do your best, persevere, and don't give up!

Be Content
We are all special in our own way. Celebrate who you are with gratitude.

We are part of something bigger than ourselves! We are part of our communities, the world, and the universe!

Adapted from Yoga for Children by Lisa Flynn

Your First Yoga Class

When beginning a new series such as "Planting Seeds" or any other curriculum, you will probably want to begin with a brief introduction of "What is Yoga?" If this is your first class with a new group of students, you will want to introduce yourself to the class and facilitate introducing themselves to each other, as well.

You may lead your own discussion or follow this one:

Opening Discussion: What is Yoga?

The word "yoga" means "union."

Question: What are we bringing together in yoga?

Possible Answers: *Breath and movement, mind and body, friends*

What we learn in yoga, we can take with us as we move throughout our day. We can use our breath to calm ourselves, we can use poses to make our bodies work well and feel good, and, most importantly, we can treat everyone like they have a special "light" inside of them, which we see and respect.

Question: Why do we practice yoga?

Possible Answers: *To help our bodies and minds relax, to calm ourselves, to be physically healthy, etc.* **Yoga is good for our brains and our bodies.**

Question: How can practicing yoga make the world a better place?

Possible Answers: *When we are feeling and doing our best, we share that energy with those around us. Treating others as we wish to be treated will make our friends and family feel happier and appreciated. Respecting others and our surroundings will help other people and keep the earth a beautiful place to live.*

Question: Where did yoga start?

Answer: Yoga began in India thousands of years ago.
Yogis began to study the world around them and learn how animals and nature worked together. They learned ways to move their bodies to be healthy, and how to make their brains strong by being **mindful**. Mindfulness is bringing concentration and focus to one thing at a time.

Yoga Class and Our Agreements

In order to have fun in yoga, we need to agree on acceptable behavior in class.

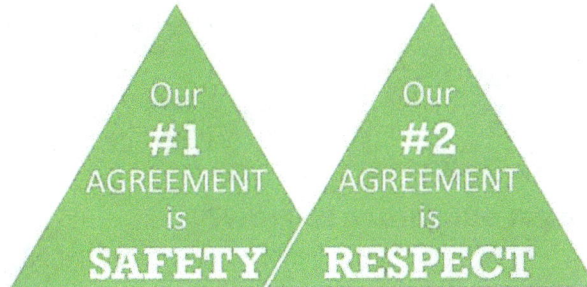

Our **#1** AGREEMENT is **SAFETY**   Our **#2** AGREEMENT is **RESPECT**

SAFETY
We try new poses together, with supervision.
We keep hands to ourselves.
We stay on our mats unless told otherwise.

RESPECT
RESPECT for OURSELVES
RESPECT for OTHERS
RESPECT for our ENVIRONMENT

This is a good time to go over other housekeeping items. Don't make the list too long. Generally, we have 2 things that should be done at the beginning or before class:

- Use the restroom
- Fill your water bottle

You can structure a routine that covers what to do when entering the yoga room (where to put their backpacks if they are coming from school, where to put their shoes, designate a place to eat their snack, etc.)

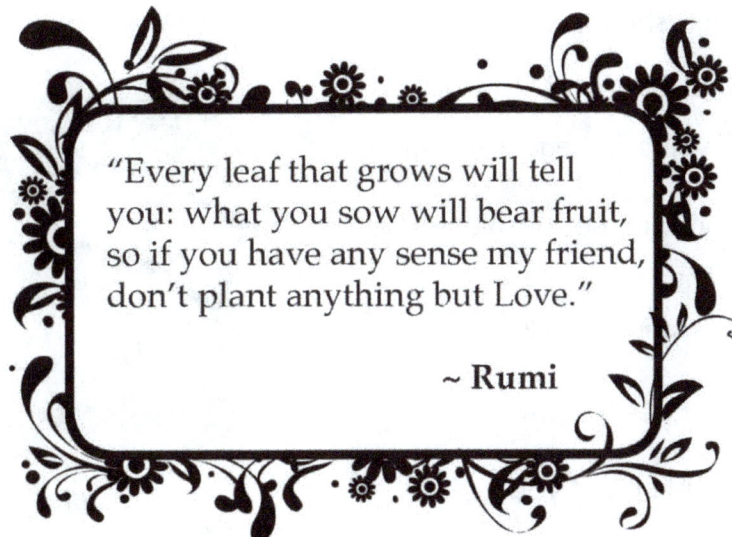

"Every leaf that grows will tell you: what you sow will bear fruit, so if you have any sense my friend, don't plant anything but Love."

~ Rumi

Planting Seeds — ONE

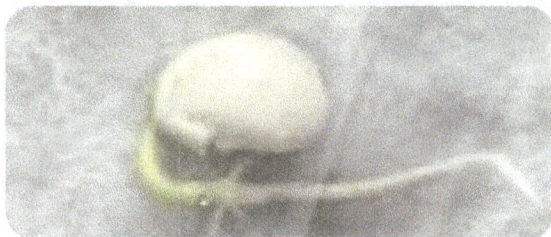

> Before classes begin, start a lima bean in a see-through bag.
>
> Check the progress of its growth on the first and third week of class (or more frequently).

Circle Time: How do we get our garden to grow?

Connection: Seeds make our garden grow!

Read: *National Geographic Readers: Seed to Plant*
By Kristin Baird Rattini

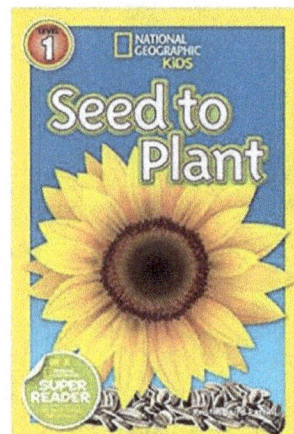

> We rarely read an entire book in yoga class. Choose a section that teaches the basics of the lesson. Books with pictures are best for little ones, of course.

Move: How a seed becomes a plant

Act this out as a group:

Begin in a crouched position, being as tiny as you can be.

Pretend you are a seed planted in the earth.

Now the sun is shining on you and you have water being poured onto you.

How does a plant grow? Slow or fast?

As slowly as you can, begin to unfurl and grow.

First, our heads pop out of the ground.

Then a leaf. Then two.

Finally, we are standing tall.

Ask: What kind of plant are you?

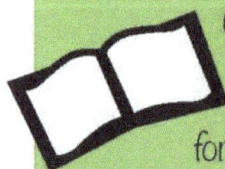

> **We Love Books!** Our lesson plans often include ideas for books, but they are just suggestions. If the books mentioned are not available or appropriate for your group, please feel free to choose alternatives.

⭐ **Affirmation:** **We have to plant a seed for something to grow!**
(We have to make an effort/take action to get a result.) ⭐

Move: **Yoga My Name**

Divide into 2 groups to play if there are lots of kids.

Have each student say their name and make the letter shapes with their body.
Everyone follows along.
Too many kids or short on time? Make the first letter of each child's name.
At the end, have everyone spell YOGA and make a chant out of it. Older kids can try
to make it similar to the song "YMCA." (See lyrics in **Resources.**)

Mindful Activity: **Seed Detective**

**Bring in a variety of plant seeds. Look at different kinds of seeds and have kids guess
what type of plant they will grow.**

Divide into 2 small groups to play if there are lots of kids.

- Take an envelope with 6 - 10 different seeds in it. Spread them out.*

- Have the whole group look at and examine all of the seeds. Notice how they are
  different and how they are the same.

- Pick one student to go first. Other students close their eyes.

- This person will mix the seeds up and take one seed out of the group.

- Place all the remaining seeds back in the middle of the circle.

- See if the group can figure out which seed is missing.

   * Make this game easier or harder depending on the ages of your children.

Game: **Play "Small Tree, Tall Tree"**

See next page.

Breath:

Take time to explain the importance of **Breath**. A good amount of the oxygen
we inhale (breathe in) is used by our brains. When we are upset or scared, our
breathing becomes short and shallow. Our thinking brain can shut down. But if we
can get some more oxygen to our brain, we can "turn it on" again and make better
choices.

Refer to Dan Seigel's "Hand Brain" for yourself. Share this video if there is time in
class and you have access to a screen. *https://www.youtube.com/watch?v=gm9CIJ74Oxw*

OMtastic Yoga

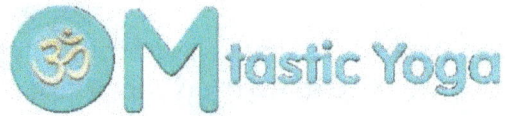

Games for School Age

TALL TREE, SMALL TREE

Materials: none, but the more space, the better

"Tall Tree, Small Tree" is a version of "Red Light, Green Light"

DIRECTIONS

Choose one student to be "It" to start the game. Everyone else lines up at the far end of the space and the person who is "It" stands with their back to the line of kids. When their back is turned, "It" says, loudly enough for all to hear: "Tall Tree Small Tree, 1, 2, 3." Then, the person who is "It" turns around to face the other children.

During the time the person who is "It" is speaking, the students in line can walk quietly toward "It" but when "It" turns around, the students must be frozen in Tree Pose.

If the person who is "It" sees anyone moving (not in Tree Pose), those people get sent back to the beginning line.

(Wobbling in Tree Pose does not count as moving.)

The first student to reach "It" and tap them gently on the back becomes "It" for the next round.

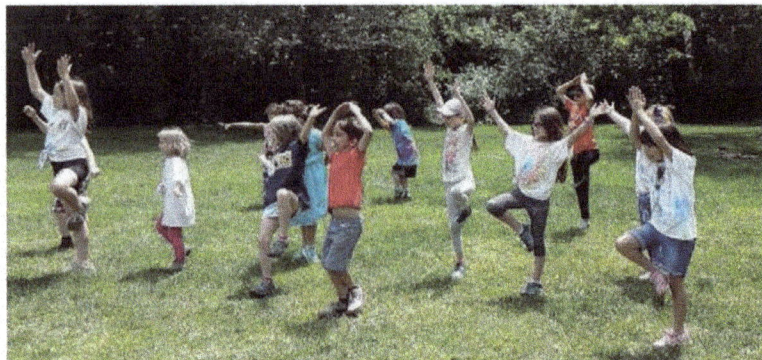

Cooling Tongue Breath:

This is a cooling breath that can be used after exercising or a day of being outside.

- Sit in a comfortable position, with your hands resting on your knees.

- If you can, curl your tongue (this is a genetic trait and not everyone will be able to do this). If you can't curl your tongue, breathe through a small opening in your mouth (like you have a straw between your lips).

- Inhale and exhale with your tongue in this position.

- Repeat 5 times.

- Notice how your body is feeling. Does your mouth feel cooler?

- Drink water after practicing this breath, as it can make your mouth dry.

Savasana:
Introduce the idea that our bodies need to rest as well as move to get strong and healthy. When our bodies rest, we can also let our minds be still from thinking all the time. Minds need rest, too.

Idea for script:

Imagine that you have been outside on a warm spring day planting in your garden.

Now it is time to rest and admire your hard work. Find a comfortable position and let your body begin to relax.

(Closing eyes and lying down are optional. Make sure kids feel comfortable and safe.)

Imagine that you are lying under a beautiful tree and you can feel the coolness of the shade on your skin.

Imagine the sun warming the earth where you just planted the seeds in your garden. As the sun warms the earth, you can see the little seeds start to grow!

As the days pass, and the sun and rain nourish your garden, your seeds burst out of the ground with stems and leaves reaching for the sky. Send warm thoughts to these new plants just beginning their lives.

Now, imagine your plants have grown tall with your care, and they are bearing fruit. Red, juicy tomatoes, green, crunchy peppers, golden-yellow squash, ripe, red strawberries, and sweet watermelon.

See yourself in the garden picking these yummy fruits and veggies, sharing them with your friends.

Take a moment to breathe in their fresh scent.

Bring your hands over your head and take a big stretch. Hug your knees to your chest and roll up to a comfortable seat.

Closing: Namasté Song

See **Resources** for closing songs

Repeat the affirmation: We have to plant a seed for something to grow!

Show kids the lima bean seed you have begun to grow. Revisit the growth as time permits during the session.

Roll up mats, clean space. Hand out coloring sheet to take home, or add into class if there is time.

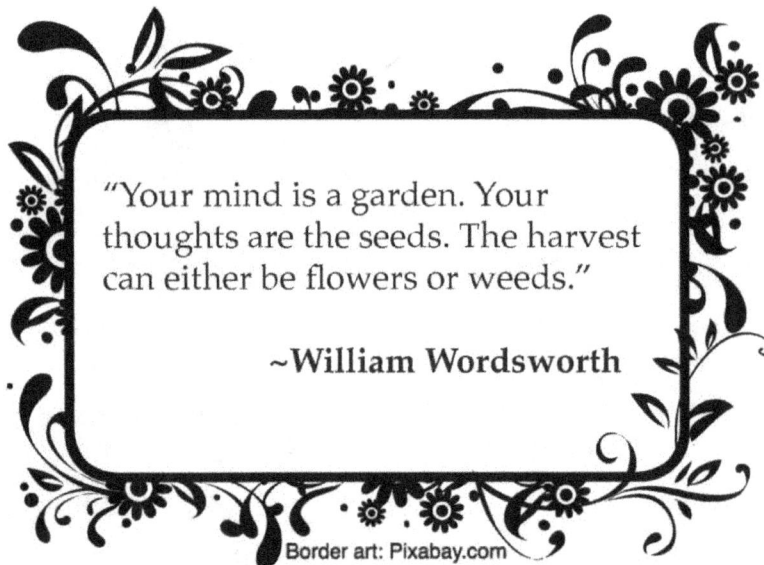

"Your mind is a garden. Your thoughts are the seeds. The harvest can either be flowers or weeds."

~William Wordsworth

Border art: Pixabay.com

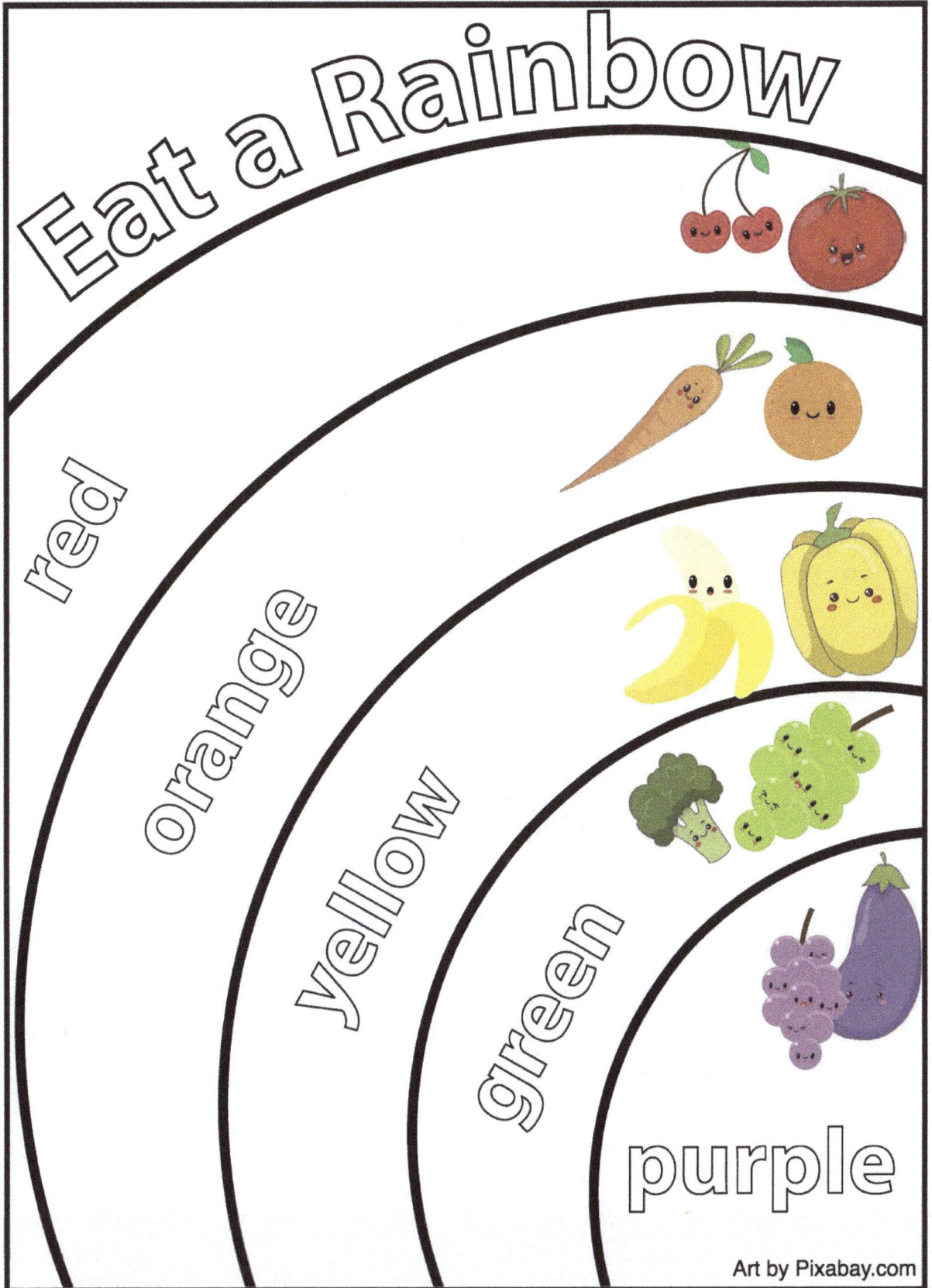

Eat a Rainbow

red

orange

yellow

green

purple

Art by Pixabay.com

BONUS LESSON ADDITION

We try to include relevant occasions and celebrations, as well as important events that occur, during our session times. For example, we always add a Fall/Halloween themed class if we are meeting in October.

Oftentimes, the Planting Seeds curriculum is offered in Spring, so Earth Day is a great time to add these activities to class – or create an entire class based on Earth Day.

Celebrating Earth Day Any Day!

Maybe Earth Day (April) is coming soon, or has happened recently. But, even if it's a long time from now, find an occasion to celebrate the Earth with a special class. Talk about recycling, reusing, and reducing. Maybe organize a clean-up project at school or wherever your classes are held.

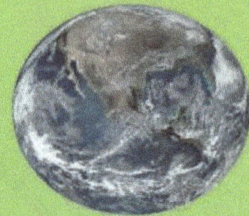

Storytime: Earth Day Story with Yoga
See **Resources** for "Earth Day Story"

Activity: Earth Day Every Day coloring sheet
Send the coloring sheet home if there wasn't enough time to work on it in class.

Closing: Share some ways to care for the earth this week.

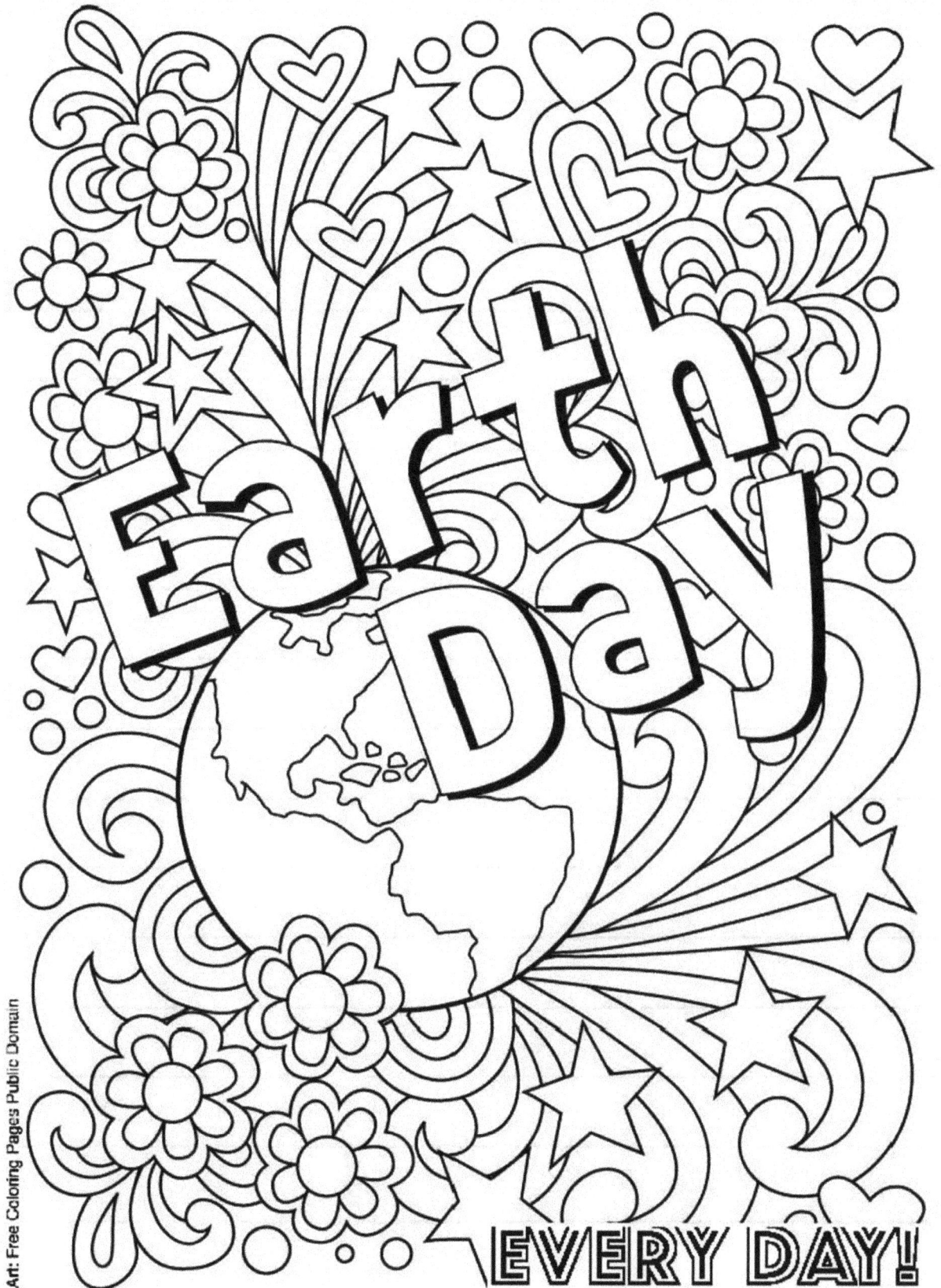

Earth Day Every Day!

Art: Free Coloring Pages Public Domain

Teacher's Notes:

_____

_____

_____

_____

_____

_____

_____

_____

_____

_____

_____

_____

_____

Teacher's Notes:

_____

_____

_____

_____

_____

_____

_____

_____

_____

_____

_____

_____

_____

_____

Planting Seeds of Gratitude & Kindness   TWO

Focus: We all need gratitude and kindness in our lives. It can make our brains learn to think happier thoughts more often.

☼ **Research Shows...**
the more often we think kind thoughts or reflect on things we are grateful for in our lives, the more our brains rewire to think happier thoughts more often!
We can become healthier and less stressed!

https://www.umassd.edu/counseling/forparents/recommendedreadings/theimportanceofgratitude/

Circle Time: Say your name and one thing you are grateful for.

Connection: Showing kindness and gratitude to others can make us feel good.

Move: Sun Salutation
See **Resources**

Read: *If You Plant a Seed* by Kadir Nelson

Do yoga poses as you read the story.

- What did the animals learn at the end of the story?
- How does this apply to you?

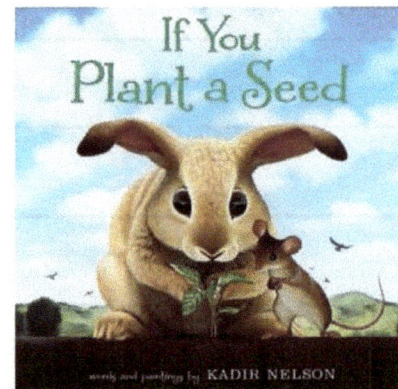

⭐   **Affirmation:**   I am kind to myself and others.   ⭐

Move: Musical Mats
- Place mats in a circle.

- Place a card with a pose (name or picture) on it in front of each mat.

- When the music starts, have the children walk around the mats.

- When the music stops, everyone must find a mat and do the pose on the card.

- You can direct the kids to hop, skip, tiptoe, jump, etc. when the music is on or let them move any way they like.

Craft: **Make a Gratitude Journal**
             See Resources

You may want to prepare the booklets ahead of time for younger kids.
Invite children to decorate their journals however they like.
They can draw or write something they are grateful for, and update each week.

Story: **"Muhammad and the Cat"** from *The Treasure in Your Heart*
             See Resources for the story.

Have the children pretend to be the cat, curled up and listening to the story.
Note that the story refers to a "prophet" named "Muhammad." If you want to
change "prophet" to "wise man" or "teacher" you can always alter stories to fit
your group.

Breath: **Back-to-Back Breathing**

•   Sit back-to-back with a partner.

•   Notice the breath of your partner and try to match your breath to theirs.

•   As you inhale, think about something you are grateful for about your partner.

•   Turn around and share your gratitude.

•   Change partners and repeat.

Mindful Activity: **Gratitude Jar**

•   Give everyone a small note card or sticky note.

•   Ask them to write one thing they are grateful for on the note.

•   Place the cards in a jar or other container.

•   Draw one card (sticky note) and read it to the group.

•   See if other people in the group are grateful for the same thing.

•   Have everyone sit for just a moment and concentrate on this "gratitude."

Closing:

Thinking of the thing you are grateful for, take a deep breath in and breathe out your word in a whisper. Bring your hands to your heart and say "Thank You" aloud or to yourself.

Keep the jar with the notes in it and share a new gratitude next week.

Keep journals (be sure their names are on them).

Roll up mats, clean up space.

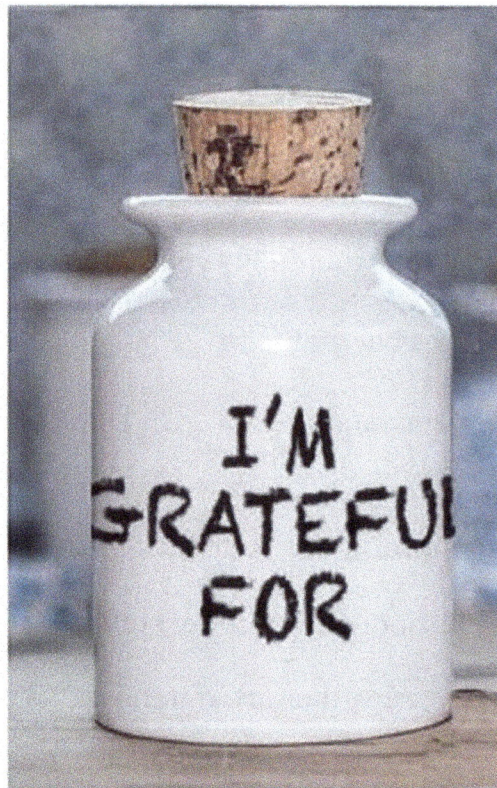

Photo: Pixabay.com

Teacher's Notes:

_____

_____

_____

_____

_____

_____

_____

_____

_____

_____

_____

_____

_____

_____

Teacher's Notes:

_____

_____

_____

_____

_____

_____

_____

_____

_____

_____

_____

_____

_____

Parts of Our Plants — THREE

Focus: Every seed grows roots, stems, and leaves.

Connection: If I care for the seed and the earth it is planted in,
my plant will grow and provide food for me.

- Have you ever worked in a garden?

- How does it feel to work outside in the dirt?

Move: **Sun Salutation**
Add on from last week

Read: *National Geographic Readers: Seed to Plant*
by Kristin Baird Rattini

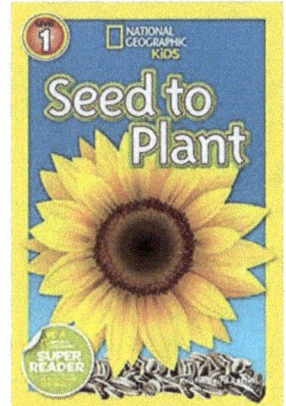

Look at the section that talks about the parts of plants.

Check on the lima bean you planted on the first week. What changes can you notice?

★ **Affirmation:**   **I can take care of my plants so they will grow.** ★

Move: **Be a Tree**

Practice being a tree!

If your weather is good, you could even do this outdoors, letting the children feel the grass and earth under their feet.

First, notice your feet. Spread your toes wide for a good strong foundation. These are your roots.

Next, move to your legs. The trunk of a tree is very strong. Only when a tree becomes sick (or maybe in a very bad storm) does its trunk move or break. Make your legs strong.

Next, move to the branches of your tree. Branches grow in many different shapes and sizes. Make your arms like branches.

What kind of tree are you?

Now, come into Tree Pose and see if you can be steady and strong like real trees.

Maybe you can be so still that you hear your breath.

Put on the song "Big Old Tree" and have kids act out the song.
David Weinstone Presents Music for Aardvarks and Other Mammals

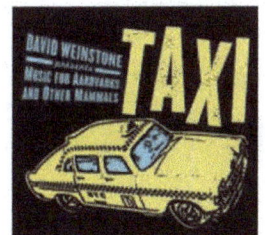

OMtastic Yoga

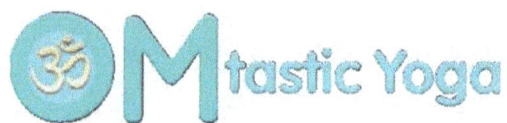

Preschool Songs

BIG OLD TREE

https://youtu.be/zKxDWE4ucPc

Great for practicing balance in Tree Pose. Encourage kids to come back into the pose after they have fallen out. Switch legs a few times.

I am a big old tree	Tree Pose
Stuck in the ground is me	Sad face in tree pose
If I had just one wish	Hold up 1 finger
I'd like to dance like this	
I'd do a little bump	Bump hips left and right
I'd do a little twist	Twist hips
I'd do a little jump	Jump
I'd wiggle just like this	Wiggle Body
I'd do the Funky Chicken	Flap wings
It's silly, yes I know	
And then I'd pack my trunk	Clap
And hit the road	Swing hitchhiking thumb behind you, over your shoulder.

Exact movements are not important. Just have fun!

Alternate Moving Activity:

We've been having a little trouble finding "Big Old Tree" recordings available on music apps, so a good alternative is "Roots, Stems, Leaves, Flowers."

Check out this great resource from Firefly Family Theater!

https:www.youtube.com/watch?v=9bFU_wJgvBIBI

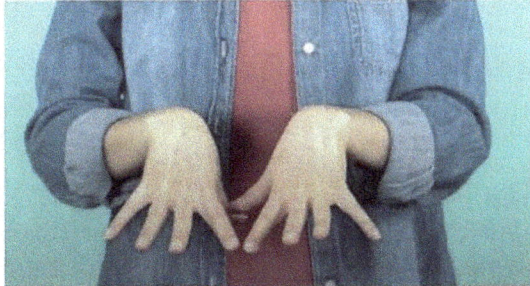

ROOTS

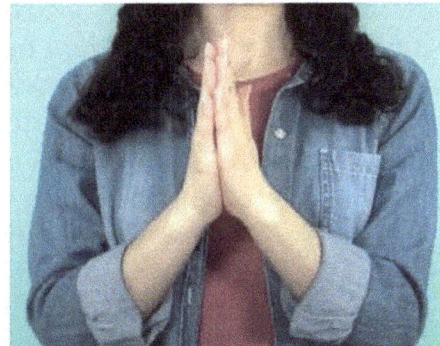

STEM

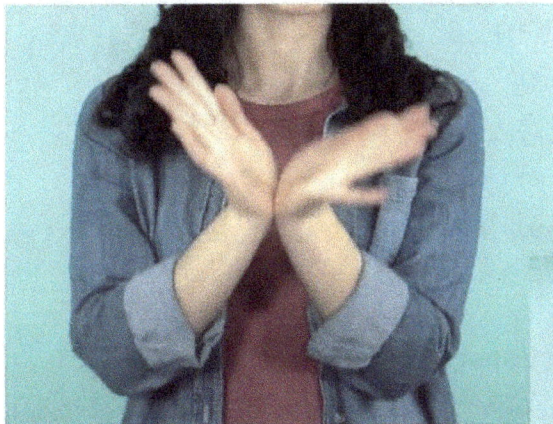

LEAVES

FLOWERS

SUN, AIR, RAIN SHOWERS

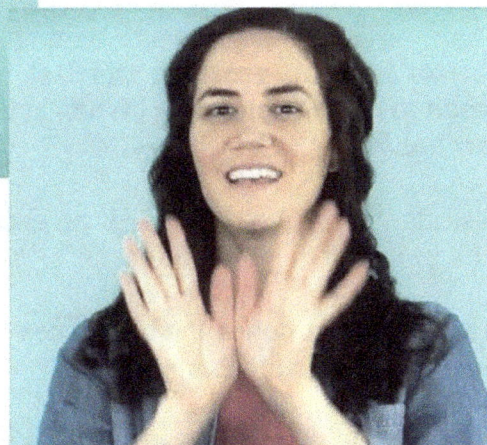

Firefly Family Theater has many more fun resources!
https://www.youtube.com/@fireflyfamilytheatre3882

Game: Rock, Tree, Bridge

- Have students get into groups of 3.

- The first student gets down in Rock Pose (Child's Pose).

- The second student steps over the rock and comes into Tree Pose.

- The third student steps over the rock, goes around the tree, and makes a bridge (Down Dog Pose).

- Now, the first person goes around the tree, under the bridge, and then becomes a rock. They are slowly moving forward with each new pose.

- Repeat until students reach the other side of the room.

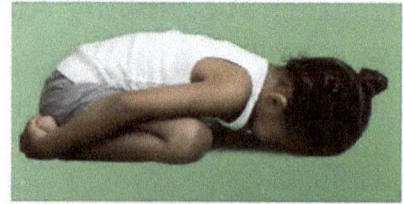

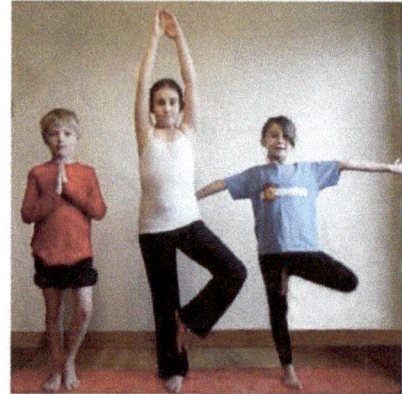

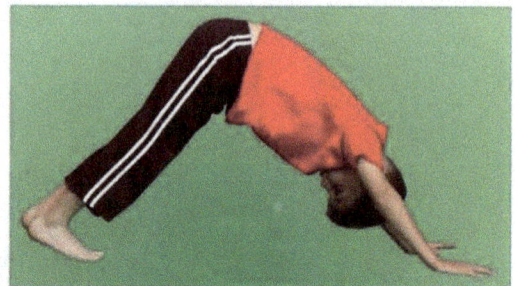

Story: "The Magic Pear Tree" (China) from *Storytime Yoga*

Breath: Staircase Breathing

Great for releasing tension, building awareness of those around you, and getting silly.

NOTE: Not a trauma-sensitive exercise!
You need to know your group. "When in doubt, leave it out."

Have students lay with their heads on each other's belly, forming a ladder.

Have each student notice the breath coming in and out of their neighbor's belly.

Then, starting with the first person, pass a "ha" down the line, then two "ha"s and then three "ha"s. By now, hopefully, there will be some laughter.

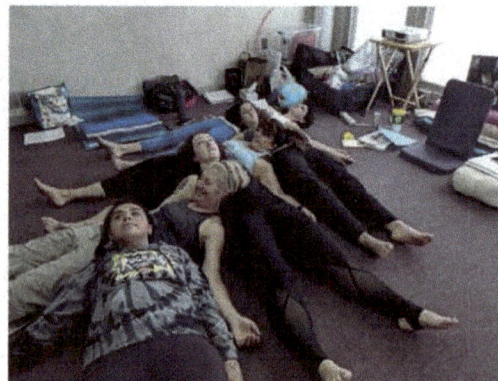

Mindful Activity: **Find a Color Game**
Come to a comfortable seat in a circle.

- Have everyone look around the room and find something that is red (or any color you choose).

- When everyone has something in mind, have them give a "Thumbs up" signal.

- Start sharing around the circle.

- Once one object has been named, no one else can name it – they must look around and find something else that color.

Flowering Plant (Angiosperm) Anatomy

Illustration: Public Domain

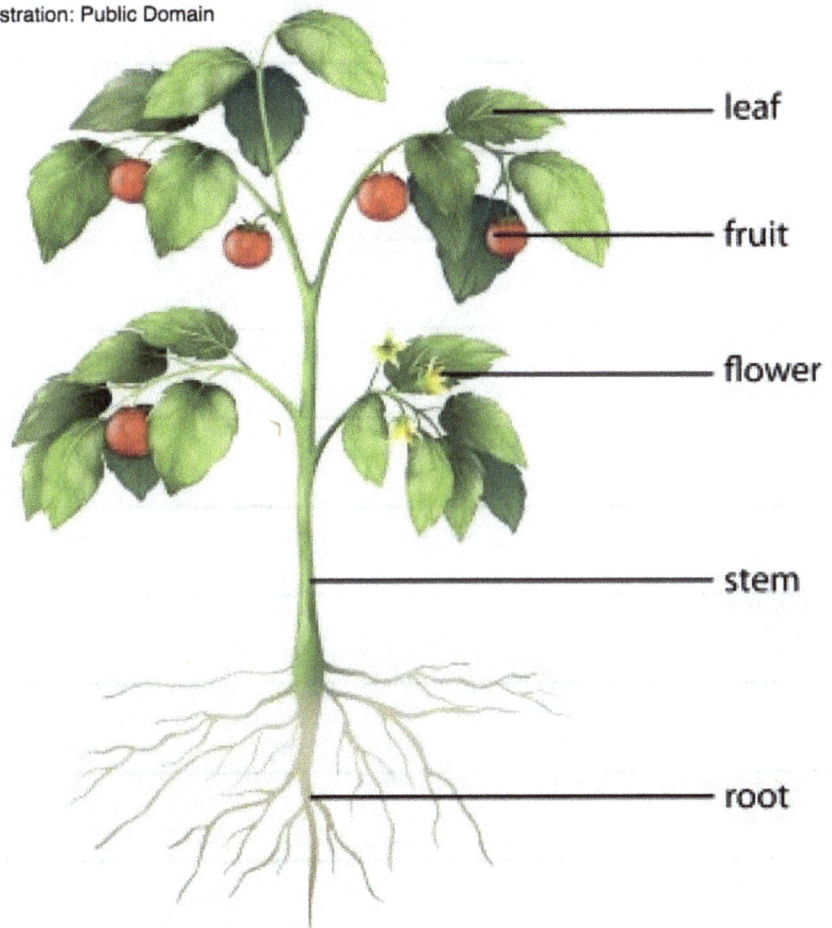

leaf

fruit

flower

stem

root

Closing:
You may want to introduce Savasana with Breathing Buddies (see **Resources**).

When Savasana is over, pull a new gratitude out and read it to the group. Ask if anyone else is grateful for this same thing. Bring hands to your heart "Namasté."

Teacher's Notes:

_____

_____

_____

_____

_____

_____

_____

_____

_____

_____

_____

_____

_____

Teacher's Notes:

_____

_____

_____

_____

_____

_____

_____

_____

_____

_____

_____

_____

_____

FOUR

Focus: What activities, people, or places make me smile?

Connection: It is important to bring joy into my life.
Think about what times are the happiest for you.

Move: Have students divide into groups of 2 or 3. Each group will have 5 minutes (or whatever you determine) to come up with a yoga routine to teach the whole class.

JOY IS CONTAGIOUS

Read: *Chrysanthemum* by Kevin Henkes

Discuss how important it is to be an individual, and that by being unique, we make the world a great place.

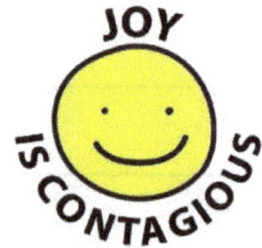

Make and color a heart map (next page). Write the names of people you love in different sections. Color these sections red. Write the names of places you love in other sections. Color them blue. Continue until your heart is filled with colors.

★ **Affirmation:** When I am happy, the people around me are happy, too! ★

Song: *My Roots Go Down*
See **Resources**

Mindful Activity:
Pass out scarfs to everyone. Ask them to pretend to be:
- Seaweed
- The wind
- The ocean
- A flower swaying in a light breeze
- A tree moving in strong wind

You can find fun music to go with each movement.

Lightweight, sheer scarves are best for "floating."

Breath: Flying Bird Breath
- Stand in Tadasana (Mountain Pose).
- As you inhale, bring your hands together above your head.
- As you exhale, bring your arms (wings) to your sides.
- For added balance challenge, do this in Airplane Pose on one leg as you "fly."

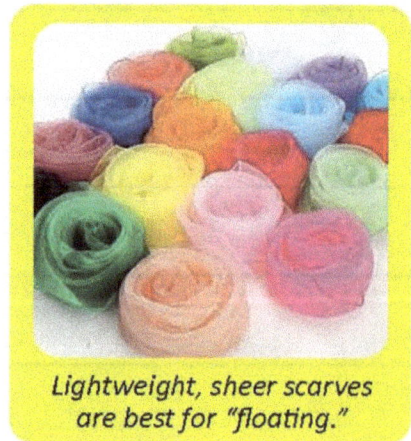

Closing: Once again, pick another gratitude to share. Be sure you pick enough each week so each child's gratitude gets shared.

Name_____ Date_____

A Few of My Favorite Things

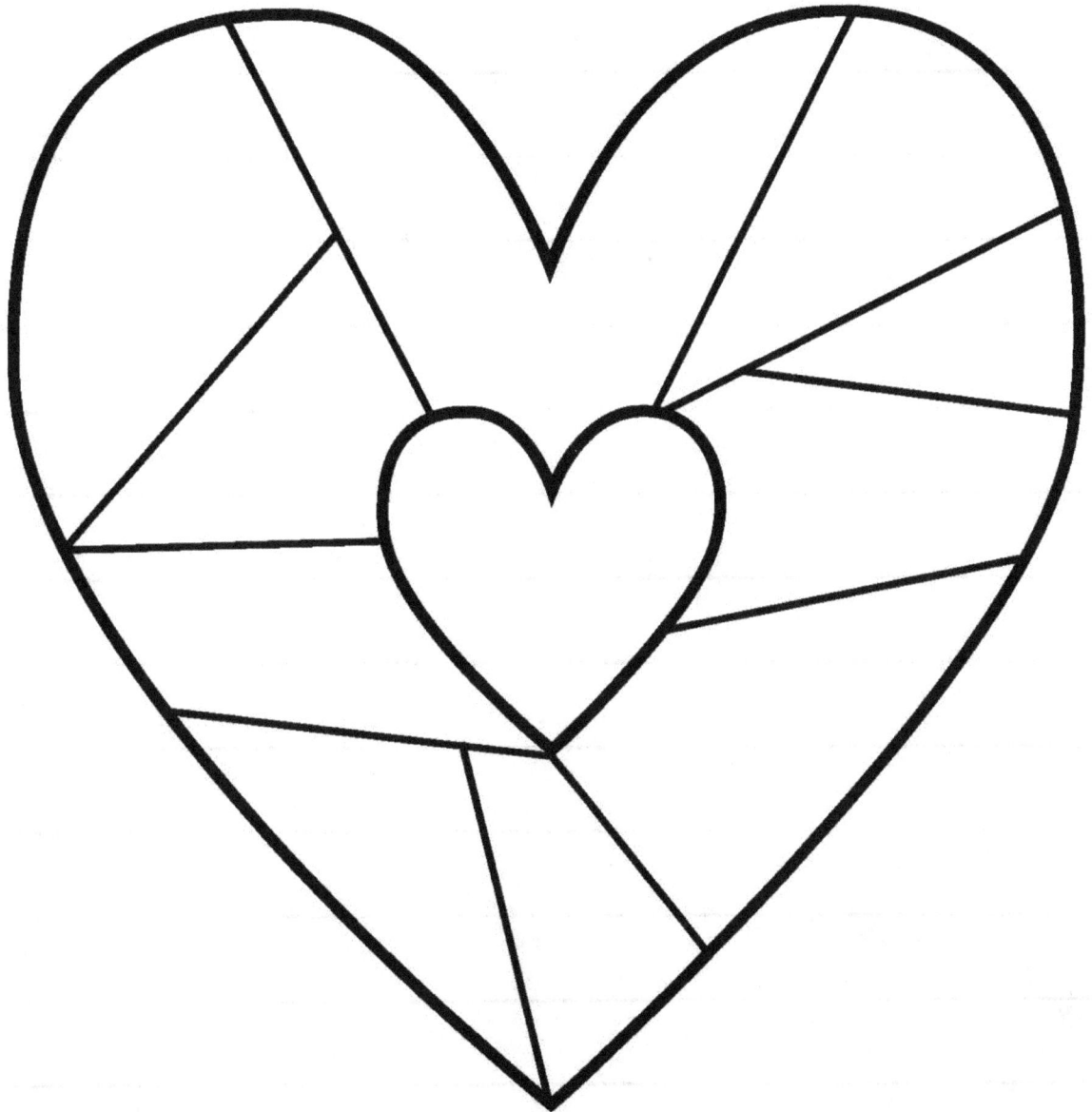

People I ♡ **Red**   **Things I** ♡ **Green**

Places I ♡ **Blue**   **Activities I** ♡ **Purple**

Teacher's Notes:

_____

_____

_____

_____

_____

_____

_____

_____

_____

_____

_____

_____

_____

_____

Teacher's Notes:

_____

_____

_____

_____

_____

_____

_____

_____

_____

_____

_____

_____

_____

The Lotus   **FIVE**

Focus: The Significance of the Lotus

Connection: Through difficulty comes growth

Circle/Discussion:

Let's come into Lotus Pose (or Easy Pose).
Today, we are going to learn about a beautiful flower called the lotus. They come in every color (show photos) and they grow in water. You may have seen water lilies in a pond. These are a form of lotus flower.

This is Lotus Mudra.

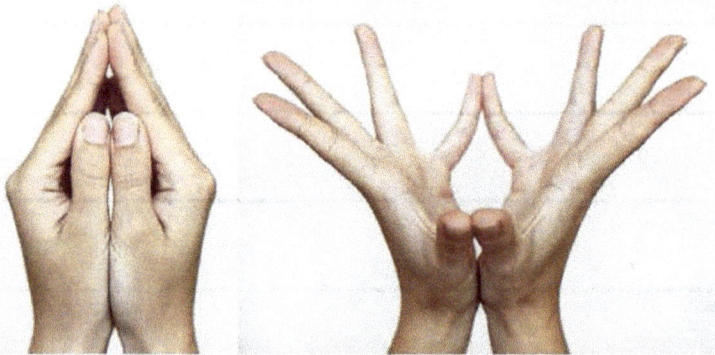

Hands face each other, palm to palm. Touch thumbs, base of palms, and pinkies to each other and open the inner fingers apart, like a blossoming flower.

What is a mudra?   Mudras can be thought of as "Yoga for your hands."

Mudras, the hand and finger gestures used in many Yoga and Ayurvedic traditions, are effective and simple tools to employ for self-soothing, energizing, settling emotions, and focusing. Like little Yoga poses for your hands, mudras make use of the energy, the prana, flowing through your body.

http://kiddingaroundyoga.com/blog/mudras-yoga-ayurveda/

What makes the lotus special is that it grows in a very muddy, murky, stagnant pond. Who knows what stagnant means? If it is stagnant, it means nothing moves out of it. So, what might be in that pond water?

Leaves *(Tree Pose)*
Dead bugs *(Dead Bug Pose)*
Worms *(Caterpillar)*
Fish *(Fish Pose)*

Kids can add ideas here.

Well, even though the conditions of the pond are not what we think of as beautiful, **guess what?** The lotus grows anyway! In fact, it actually NEEDS this stuff to grow beautiful. We might call the pond icky or gross, but it is PERFECT for the lotus to grow and thrive.

Move:
So it starts out as a tiny seed *(Child's Pose).*
And it starts to open up and grow *(rise up).*
It grows a long, strong stem that is very hard to break, it's so hard and strong *(stand stiff).*
And it pushes through the thick muddy water *(Mountain Pose).*
And finally, at the top on the water, it blooms into a beautiful flower *(Lotus Mudra)*!

For many people, the lotus is seen as very special. We can compare the lotus to our lives. Things happen in our lives that are sad, right? And some things we feel are very unfair, can be very difficult.

And YET...maybe we are strong and beautiful BECAUSE of these difficulties.

The lotus reminds us that we can be strong and try to accept these difficulties in our lives, and use them to grow into the beautiful people we are.

There is a saying, "No mud, no lotus." Can you see why this makes sense?

Breath: Flower Breath

Sit in Lotus or Easy Pose with hands on legs, palms face up. Bring fingertips and thumb tip together on each hand, as though you are holding something special in your hand.

Inhale deeply and stretch your fingers away from each other, opening your palms.

Exhale and close your fingers together (like petals of a flower closing for the evening).

Repeat 5 or so times.

Sun Salutations (add on with more advanced additions)

Mindful Activity: Lotus (leave about 20 minutes for this activity)

See **Resources** for templates and further instructions. This activity takes some time and preparation, but kids enjoy it.

We will make a lotus today, and we can keep it to remind ourselves of the things in our lives that we have to be grateful for. (Have a sample of the completed lotus to show.)

First, take 9 petals. Write a word on each of them that is something you are grateful for (or draw a picture. Something you can be happy about when you feel sad. Something that makes you feel safe when you do not feel so safe.

The first 4 words can be things you are grateful for in yourself. Maybe you are strong, funny, or kind.

The next 5 can be things outside of yourself you are grateful for. Maybe your family, friends, teachers, your home, your pet, etc.

Now, we will help you make your lotus. Lay the 4 petals side by side.
Lay the other 5 side by side.

We will tape or staple them together and set them on the lily pad.

Keep this at home to remember all that we have to be thankful for.

See **Resources** for detail and templates. View an instructional video here:
https://youtu.be/cuh1V94bvoA?si=5PsAyNqV6_wXYxVJ

Active Affirmation
In a circle:

I am happy, (hands heart center)
I am strong, (arms out flex muscles)
I am loved, (hug yourself)
and I belong! (reach out to your neighbor)

Closing:
Choose a gratitude from the jar.
Breathing Buddies or Savasana (depending on time).

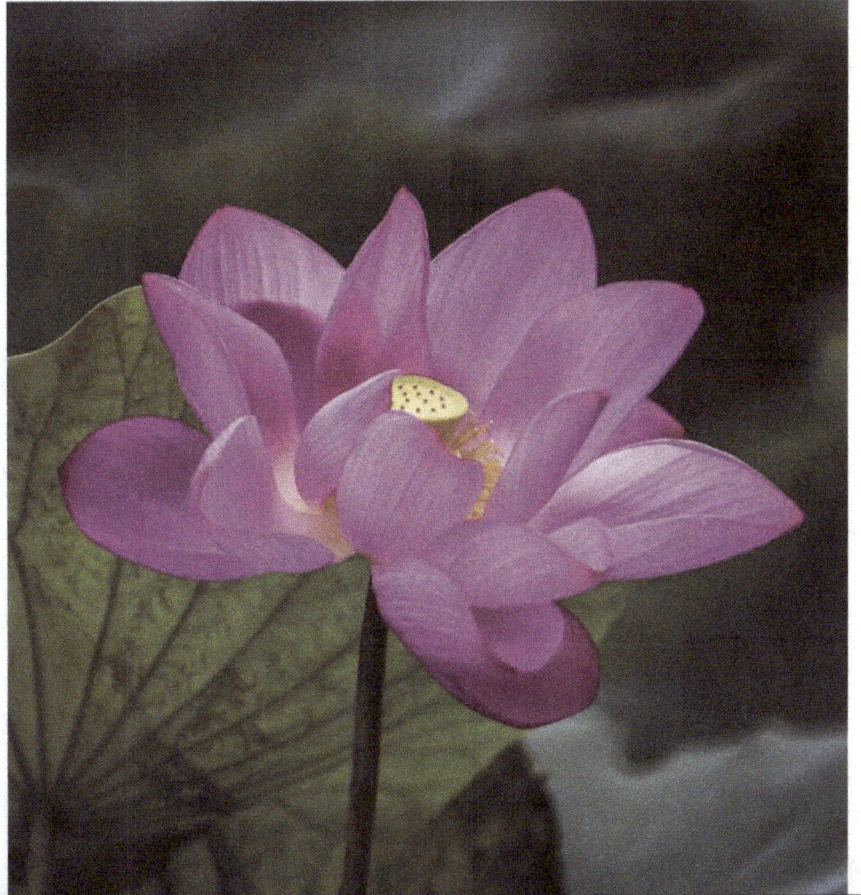

All Lotus Photos:
Pixabay.com

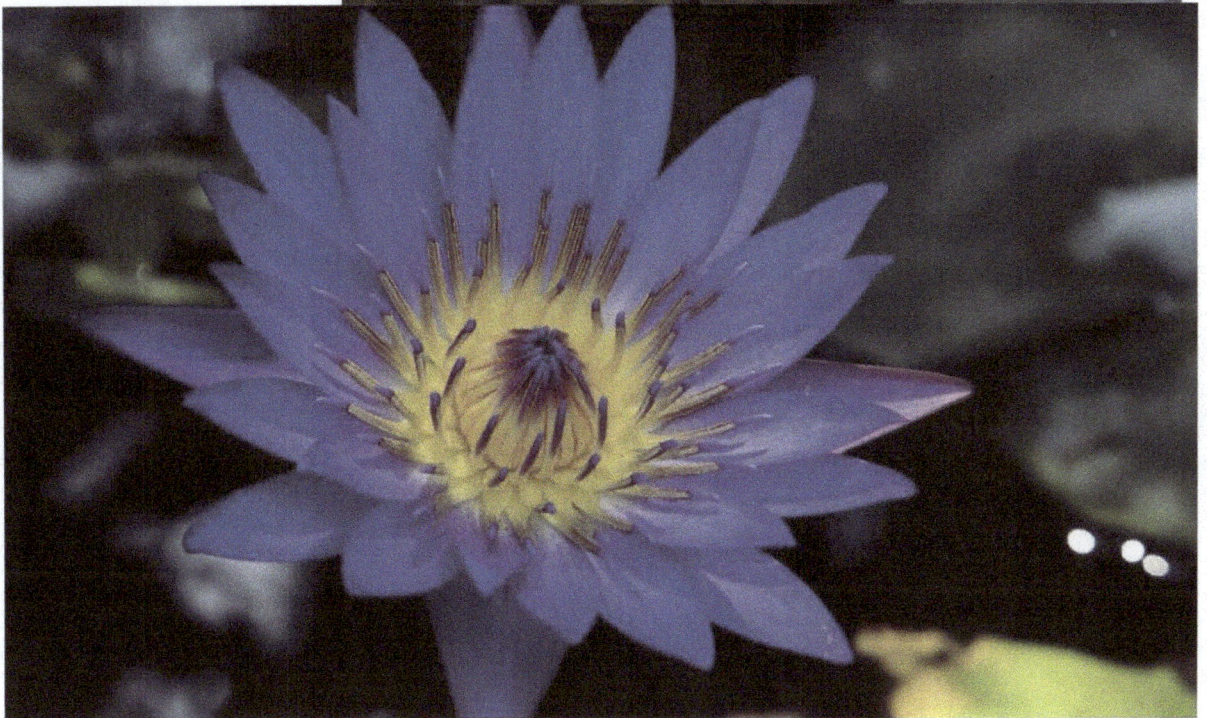

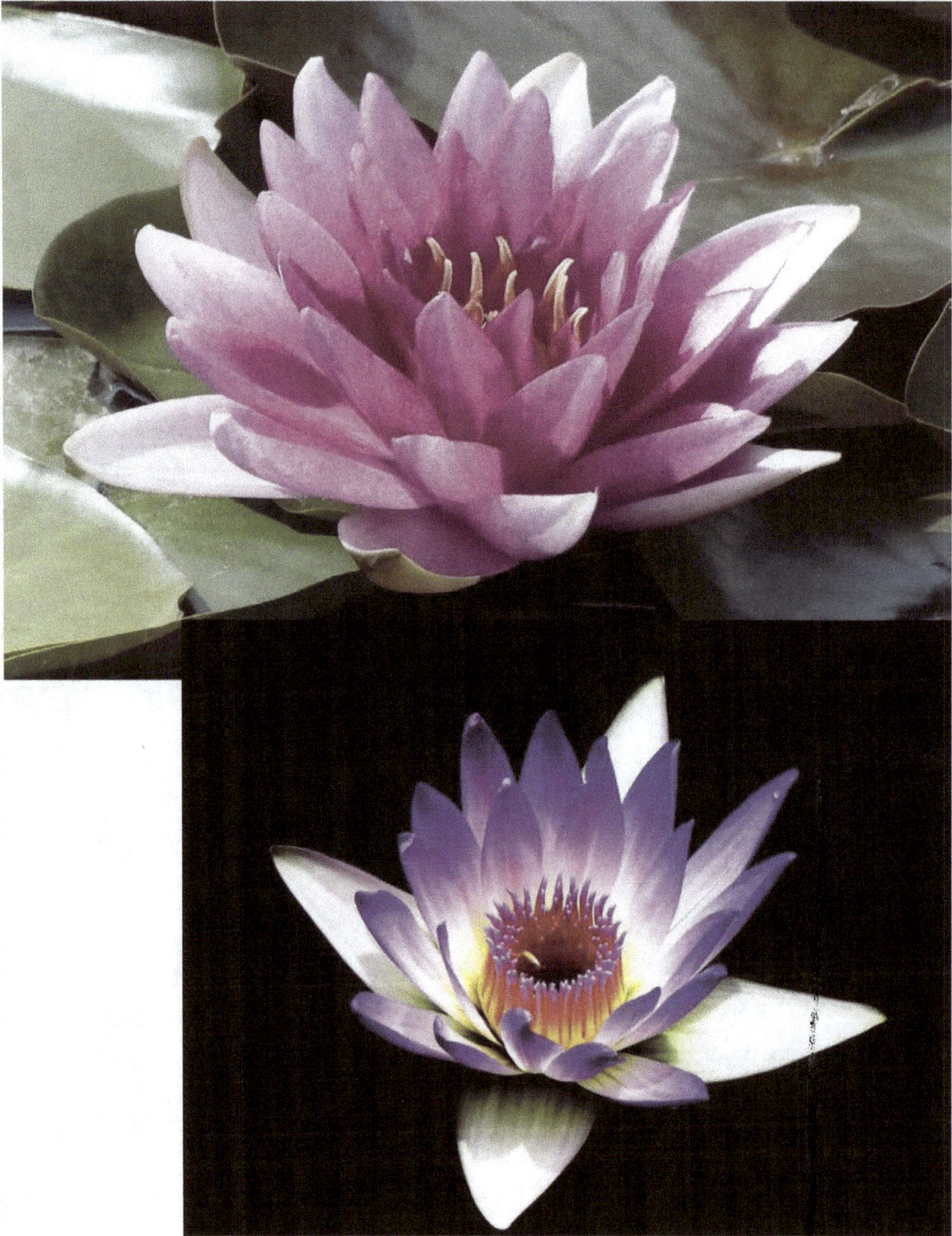

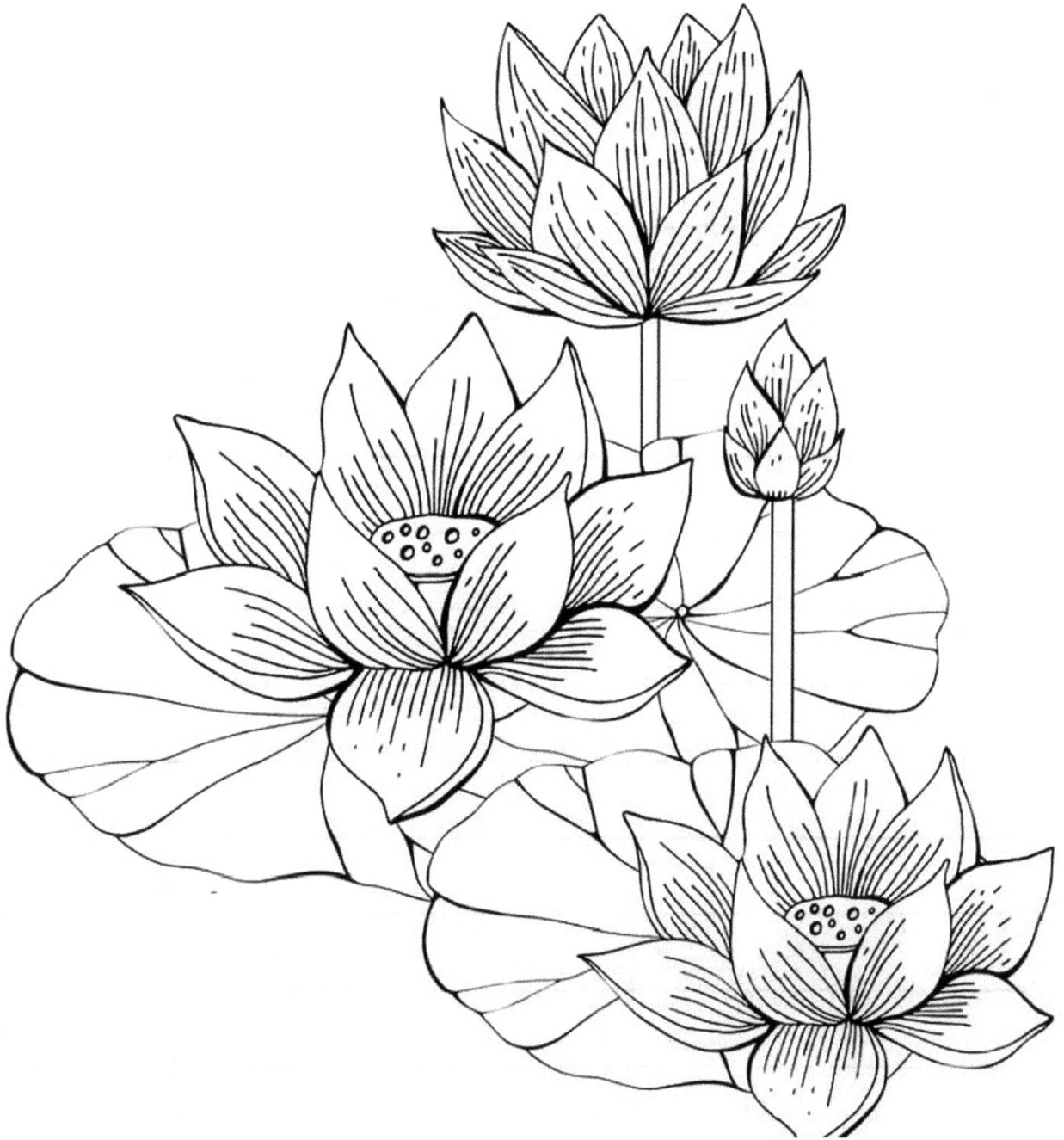

Illustration: Public Domain

The lotus flower grows out of the mud and sediment at the bottom of the pond. Without all that murky stuff, the seed would not survive.
It grows through the water into the clean air and becomes a beautiful blossom. All people experience unpleasant and sad things in their lives, and we hopefully overcome them and look back, grateful for even those **difficult times we endured.**

Teacher's Notes:

_____

_____

_____

_____

_____

_____

_____

_____

_____

_____

_____

_____

_____

Teacher's Notes:

_____

_____

_____

_____

_____

_____

_____

_____

_____

_____

_____

_____

_____

How Does Your Garden Grow?   SIX

Bring paper cups, soil, and seeds to the last class. If you can go outside to plant your seeds, it will be less messy.

Focus: **With care you can grow what you need.**

Connection: **What are your favorite fruits and vegetables?**
- How are they good for your body?
- What foods do you need to be healthy?

Read: *National Geographic: Seed to Plant*

Finish with the harvests of food.
Discuss the many steps it takes to bring food from the farm to the table.

Example: A farmer plants a seed
Farm workers tend the crops
Harvest
Put on trucks (truck driver)
Deliver to market
Store workers put out in displays
Cashier sells to you
You prepare and serve

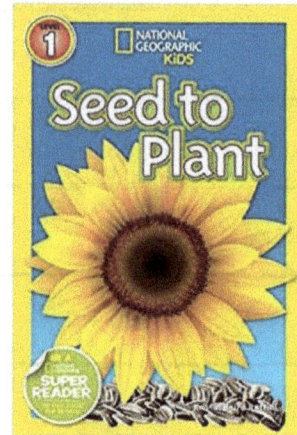

Activity: **Plant a seed in a pot to take home.**

⭐   **Affirmation:**   **My body works best when I take good care of it.**   ⭐

Planting the right seeds (eating good food, practicing mindfulness and gratitude, exercising, sleeping enough and drinking plenty of water) will grow the things I need in my life.

Move: **Do a series of poses and notice how your body changes:**

- 10 Froggy Jumps
- 10 Star to Mountain Jumps
- 3 Sun Salutations
- 10 Windmills
- Rest in Savasana after each set of poses (continued on next page).

Notice: How does your breath change?
How does your heart rate change?
What happens to your body in Savasana?
What foods give your body the fuel it needs?

Game: Make up a Story (with movement)

- Choose someone to start the game "Once upon a time."
- After the person has given their line, the group acts it out with poses.
- As you go around the circle, each person adds one line to the story, with the class acting out the story before moving to the next person.

Breath: Alternate Nostril Breath
Great for balancing both sides of your brain.

- Sit tall in a comfortable seat.
- Use one finger to close off your left nostril.
- Breathe in through the right nostril.
- Close off the right nostril and breathe out through the left.
- Keep the left open and breath in through it.
- Close the left and breathe out through the right.
- Repeat 3 times on each side.

Read: *Last Stop on Market Street* by Matt de la Peña and Christian Robinson
Discuss how it is often our perspective (the way we see things) that affects how we feel.

Mindful Activity: Mindful Eating (CHECK FOR ALLERGIES and permission)
Let everyone know that you are going to do a tasting experiment and that it works best if everyone can sit very quietly, follow directions, and use their senses of taste, touch, and smell.

- Wash your hands.
- Sit in a circle, close your eyes, and hold out your hands
- Place one slice of Mandarin Orange in everyone's hand.
- Have everyone smell the fruit.
- Have everyone notice how the fruit feels in their hands.
- Now, have everyone take a bite of the fruit but do not chew or swallow it.
- How does it taste on your tongue? How does it feel in your mouth?
- Begin to chew the fruit but don't swallow it yet. Just give it time to begin to dissolve in your mouth.
- How does it taste in your mouth? How does it feel in your mouth?
- Finally, swallow the fruit, and then sit quietly and think about all the steps it took for that food to make it to your hands and mouth to nourish your body.

Closing: Pick out one last gratitude and share it with the group!

Repeat the Affirmation:

My body works best when I take good care of it.

Planting the right seeds will grow the right things I need in my life - healthy food, and a positive attitude.

Hand out plants and containers, gratitude journals, any other items they created.

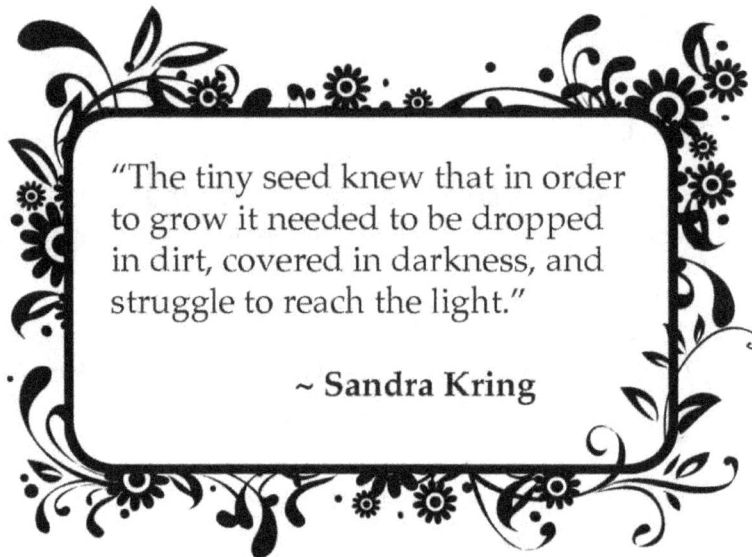

"The tiny seed knew that in order to grow it needed to be dropped in dirt, covered in darkness, and struggle to reach the light."

~ Sandra Kring

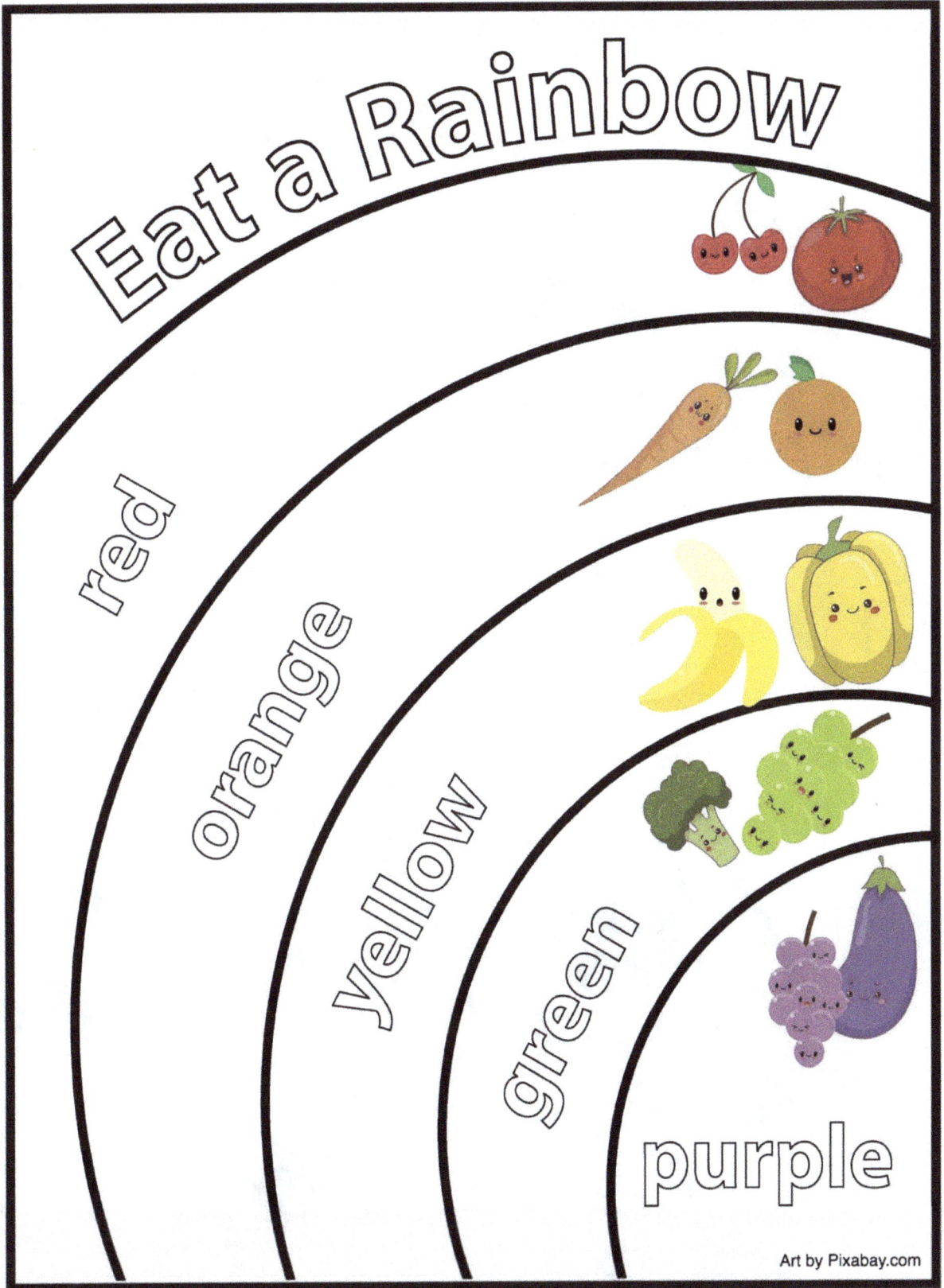

Eat a Rainbow

red

orange

yellow

green

purple

Eat a Rainbow!
(every day)

Red

Orange

Yellow

Green

Purple

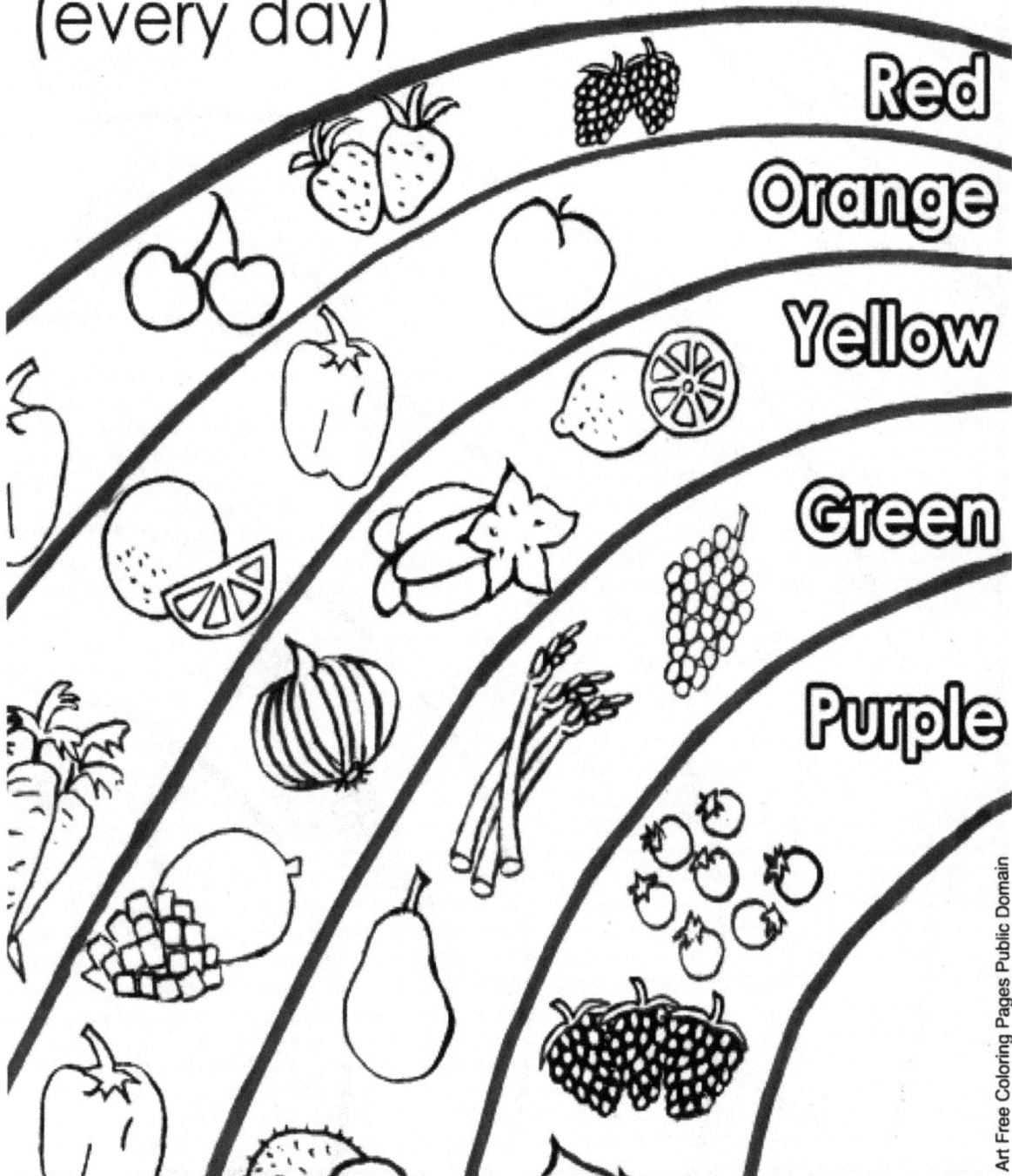

Teacher's Notes:

_____

_____

_____

_____

_____

_____

_____

_____

_____

_____

_____

_____

_____

_____

Teacher's Notes:

_____

_____

_____

_____

_____

_____

_____

_____

_____

_____

_____

_____

_____

RESOURCES

Educational Web Sites
https://www.kidsgardening.org/

Background info on seed growth
https://www.kidsgardening.org/lesson-plans-journey-to-the-center-of-a-seed/

Books

Storytime Yoga
by Sydney Solis

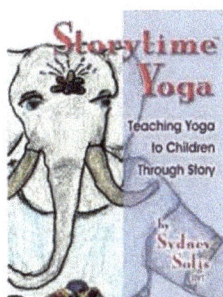

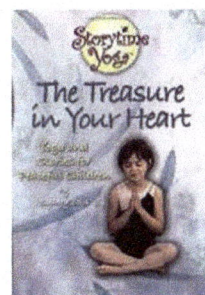

The Treasure in Your Heart
by Sydney Solis

Yoga Song to YMCA tune

Young kids, there's no need to feel down *(Forward Fold)*
I said young kids, pick yourself off the ground *(Mountain Pose)*
I said young kids, 'cause you're in a new class *(Star Pose)*
There's no need to be unhappy *(make an unhappy face)*

Young kids, there's a place you can go *(marching)*
I said young kids, when your short on your "Crow" *(Crow Pose)*
You can stay here *(standing Half Moon wave)*
And I'm sure you will find
Many ways to have a good time *(point at every one)*

> "Y-O-G-A"   It's fun to play and do"Y-O-G-A"

> They have games you can play *(hands on shoulders and walk in a circle)*
> You can learn a new pose *(Airplane Pose)*
> And hang out with all your friends *(high fives)*
> "Y-O-G-A"
> "Y-O-G-A"

Repeat until it feels done or have kids make up new verses.

There is a version of this song with no lyrics, if you want to play it in the background. It takes a little practice, but once you and the kids know it, they may ask for it again!

http://www.karaoke-version.com/mp3-backingtrack/village-people/y-m-c-a.html

Earth Day Yoga Story
by Autumn Morrison

Butterflies

Today we are going to start our adventure as butterflies *(Butterfly Pose)*. Think for a moment what kind of butterfly you would like to be: pink, orange, cabbage, painted lady? (Talk for a moment about butterflies as you "flap" your wings. What do butterflies do? They pollinate. Sip your nectar (forward bend toward your feet.

It is a beautiful spring day, birds are singing *(Bird Pose aka Airplane)*, bees are buzzing *(Bee Breath/Buzz)*. Do you know who else are pollinators? Bees!

What a beautiful day! *(Deep breath)*

All of a sudden, a human comes stomping by *(stand up, marching feet)*. Do you know what that human did? That human just picked one of the flowers from our garden and threw a piece of trash on the ground!

OOO NOOOO! That wasn't very nice of the human, was it? But what can we do about it? We're just little butterflies.

I know, let's try to talk to the human and try to teach him a better way. What do you think? *(Butterfly Pose.)* Let's fly after that human. Landing on the human's shoulder, we give a little butterfly kiss *(Kissing Pose - Lean forward on tiptoes in Airplane Pose. Blow kiss)*.

Oh, did I forget to tell you we are magic butterflies? Now, magically, the human turns into a butterfly, too! *(Butterfly Pose)*
We say, "That wasn't very nice to pick our flowers and throw away trash in our home." *(Flower Pose)*

The human is so surprised! *(Give a good surprised look.)*

"Well," he says, "I didn't think it was hurting anyone." We say, "Let us show you who you could hurt by not taking care of the environment."

So, up we fly in a forest full of trees *(Tree Pose.* As we fly, we see many trees (what kind of tree are you?

Now we see beautiful wildflowers *(Flower Pose)* and deer *(Deer Pose)*.

Flying higher, we see the green grass and mountains *(Mountain Pose)*.

Just look at how beautiful the earth is when we take care of it. Soaring over us is an eagle *(Eagle Pose)*. Down below us we see wind turbines *(Windmill Pose)*.

We come to the end of the land where the ocean begins, fed by a beautiful waterfall *(Waterfall Pose)*. A stork is trying to catch fish on the beach *(Stork Pose)* but the fish are clever and swim away *(Fish Pose)*. Oooh! Be careful, little fish, here comes a huge whale *(Whale Tail Pose)*. Let's sit for a moment and listen to the ocean *(Ocean Breath)*.

 It's a shame we can't stay here longer, but there is so much to see. So, we fly on *(Butterfly Pose)*. Soon, we come to a farm. Let's talk to that farmer over there plowing his fields *(Plow Pose)*. Excuse us, Mr. Farmer, how do you take care of the earth? "Well," says the farmer, "I never use chemicals on my crops that can harm other living beings, like bees or birds, or other humans. I only use what I need, and I always compost *(stir the compost)*.

I know, let us help the farmer add things to his compost *(still stirring)*. What can you put in compost? (Let the children come up with ideas, establishing what REALLY goes into a compost.)

"Oh, and one more thing. I recycle too," says the farmer. *(Staff Pose and stretch)*. Let's add things to the recycling. What can we put in the recycling? (Again, asking the children what is recyclable.)

I see the sun going down. Perhaps it's time to turn our friend back into a human. First, let's fly back home to our garden *(Butterfly Pose)*. Landing in our garden, we kiss our human friend *(Kissing Pose)* and *POP*! He's human again.

"Now do you see why we should take care of the earth?" we ask.

"YES!" says the human. I'm going home right now to start my compost and pick up my trash." And off he goes as we wave goodbye with our wings.

WOW that was quite an adventure!

Stork

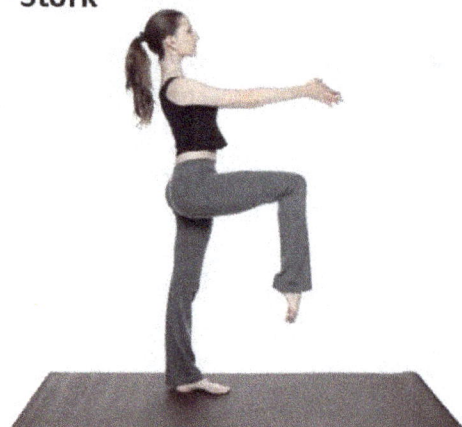

I'm sleepy, how about you?

Let's come lie down on our mats.
(Hug legs into chest one at a time then both).
Let's become a cocoon.

(Squeeze tight, then release).

Namasté Songs

You can begin or close classes with "Namasté," a Sanskrit word - a language used a long time ago in India. While many western yoga teachers use this word as a closing, it is actually a greeting (hello) in India. It means "I bow to you." If we believe there is a special light inside each of us, when we say "NAMASTÉ" we are recognizing that perfect light in the other person.

Sing "My Little Light" to the tune of "Wheels on the Bus"

My little light bows to your little light, your little light, your little light.
My little light bows to your little light, Namasté

Or

Namasté Song 2 by Kira Willey
https://www.youtube.com/watch?v=NRYaMPwJECI

The light in me sees the light in you,
The light in me sees the light in you,
I honor you as you honor me,
Namasté, Namasté, Namasté.

Or

Long Time Sun
https://www.youtube.com/watch?v=i5dRRhASY7c

May the long time sun shine upon you
All love surround you
And the pure light within you
Guide your way on.

Or

Shoshoni Namasté
https://www.youtube.com/watch?v=mK_iwaqLSyw
Namasté, Namasté,
in my heart I am grateful for you today,
Namasté, Namasté, Namasté.

The light in me
is happy to see
the light in you
shining through
Namasté, Namasté, Namasté.

GRATITUDE JOURNALS

CONSTRUCTION PAPER

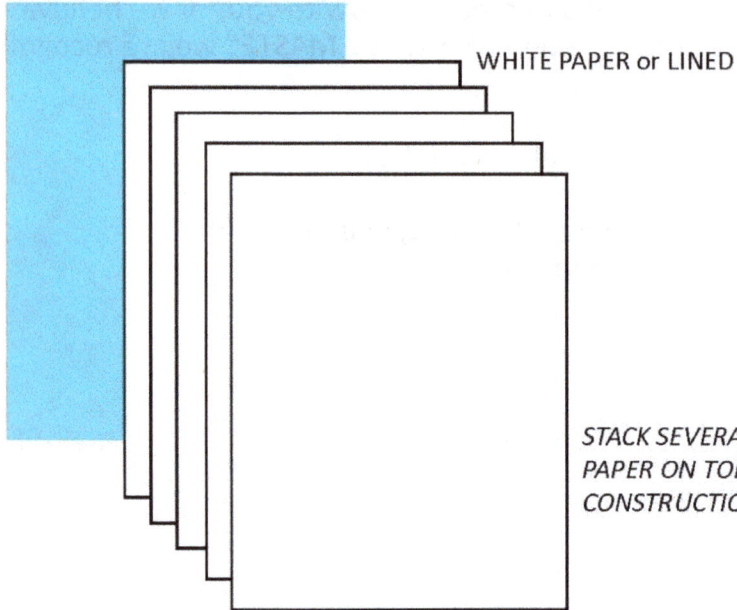

WHITE PAPER or LINED

STACK SEVERAL PIECES OF WHITE PAPER ON TOP OF ONE PIECE OF CONSTRUCTION PAPER.

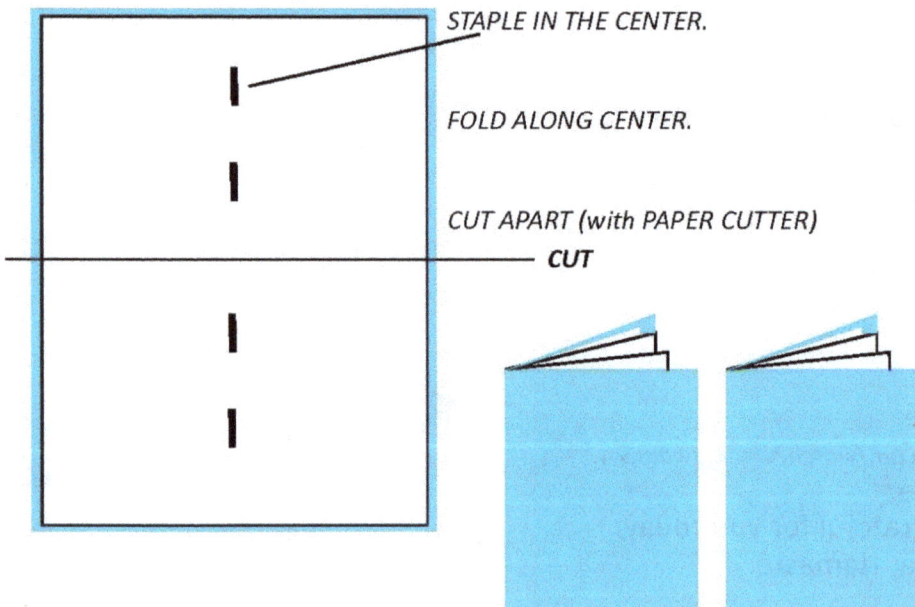

STAPLE IN THE CENTER.

FOLD ALONG CENTER.

CUT APART (with PAPER CUTTER)

CUT

KIDS CAN DECO-RATE THEIR COVERS WITH ARTWORK.

Each week, students can write and/or draw things they are grateful for.

Teaching Tales: When the Cat Came to Muhammad

From Beliefnet.com:

A traditional Muslim tale of making sacrifices to help those in need.
Stories connect us to the time-tested wisdom of the world's peoples--and teach spiritual and moral lessons we want to pass on to our kids. Each week, Beliefnet will present a spiritual story from a different faith tradition, followed by simple activities that bring the message home. We invite you to share the stories with your children, do the activities together, and make "Teaching Tales" a joyous part of family life.

One version of this very old story can be found here:
https://www.beliefnet.com/love-family/2000/09/teaching-tales-when-the-cat-came-to-muhammad.aspx

Another version is in Sydney Solis' book (see **Resources**).

Read one of these versions to the class.

Bringing It Home

To Do This Week:

Draw or paint a picture of Muhammad's wonderful robe, and then draw or paint a picture of the cat at the end of the day.

What would you do when the sick cat walked up to you? Pretend you are one of the people listening to the holy prophet. What would you do when the cat sat on his robe?

Share a story about when you asked somebody to help you. Have you ever sacrificed something to help a friend? Share a story about when a person or an animal needed your help.

Think and talk about a way to help someone in your neighborhood or school.

Sun Salutations

There are lots of good Sun Salutation songs and poems. Here is one.

FUN SUN SALUTATION IDEA

I greet the sun (MOUNTAIN) tadasana (ta-da-sa-na)

I touch the ground (FORWARD FOLD) uttanasana (oo-ta-na-sa-na)

I take big steps (PLANK)   I lower down (LOW PLANK)

I hiss like a snake (COBRA) bhujangasana (boo-jan-ga-sa-na)

I stretch like a dog (DOWN DOG) ahdo mukha svanasana (ah-doh moo-ka shva-na-sa-na)

I step over the lake (HANDS TO FEET)

I squat like a frog (FROG) malasana (ma-la-sa-na)

I reach to the sky (MOUNTAIN)

and to the sun I say (SPIN AROUND ONE TIME)

"Thanks for another beautiful day!"
(HANDS TO HEART CENTER) anjali mudra (ahn-ja-lee moo-dra)

You can add the Sanskrit names for the poses, if the kids are interested in trying to pronounce them. Explain that this is the original language of yoga!
http://www.yogajournal.com/pose-finder/

Another fun sun salutation from *StorytimeYoga.com*. Many more great stories and ideas are on Sydney's website!

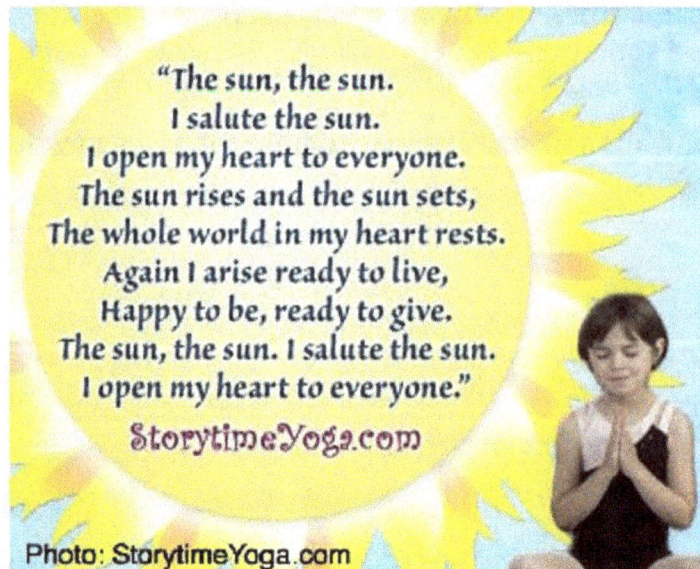

"The sun, the sun.
I salute the sun.
I open my heart to everyone.
The sun rises and the sun sets,
The whole world in my heart rests.
Again I arise ready to live,
Happy to be, ready to give.
The sun, the sun. I salute the sun.
I open my heart to everyone."

StorytimeYoga.com

Photo: StorytimeYoga.com

My Roots Go Down

words and music by Sarah Pirtle, © 1979 and 1989 Discovery Center Music BMI

Location: Two Hands Hold the Earth, Linking Up and Green Flame

Chorus:

My roots go down, down to the earth.
My roots go down, down to the earth.
My roots go down, down to the earth.
My roots go down.

Many new verses have been created:

* I am a pine tree on a mountainside.
* I am a wildflower blowing in the wind.
* I am a mountain strong and still.
* I am a willow swaying in a storm.
* I am a waterfall skipping home.
* I am a wildflower pushing through stones.
* I am a dolphin leaping high.

*The last verse sing: "From me to you, lador vador."
It is the Hebrew phrase meaning "from generation to generation."

https://www.youtube.com/watch?v=5d6jyI2dIV0

https://www.youtube.com/watch?v=dYFsbxdaJSg

Lotus Activity

You will need:

construction paper
staplers and tape
scissors
markers
templates to trace petals and lily pads

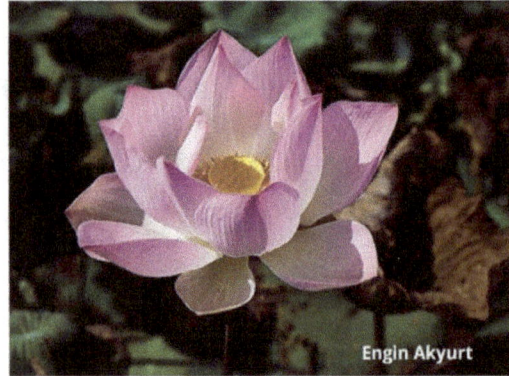
Engin Akyurt
Pixabay.com

With small kids (or large classes) you will want to cut out the petals and lily pads before class and hand them out. Older kids can trace and cut their own.

If you want to make the colors simpler (for less problems in choosing their colors), you can make all the lotus flowers multi-colored (different colors for the petals) or bring all one color paper for the petals.

First, cut out (or hand out) your lily pads. This is where your lotus will sit.

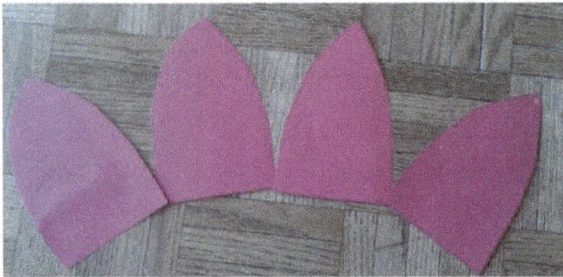

Trace and cut petals (9 for each child.)

Place 4 petals side by side in a slight arch, rather than a straight line.

Connect (glue, tape, or staple) petals at the bottom and form a ring.

Repeat with the 5 petals, making a slightly larger ring to place outside the inner ring.

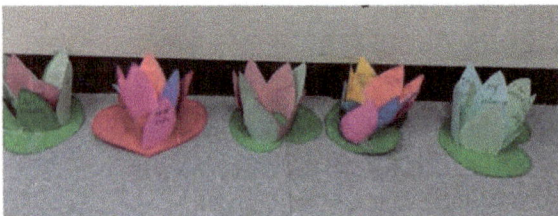

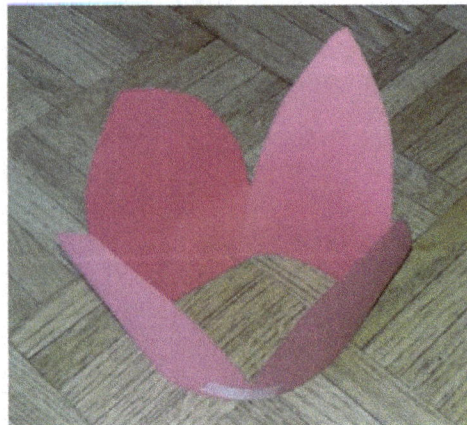

Link to YouTube Video here:
https://youtu.be/faybw3UHnIE

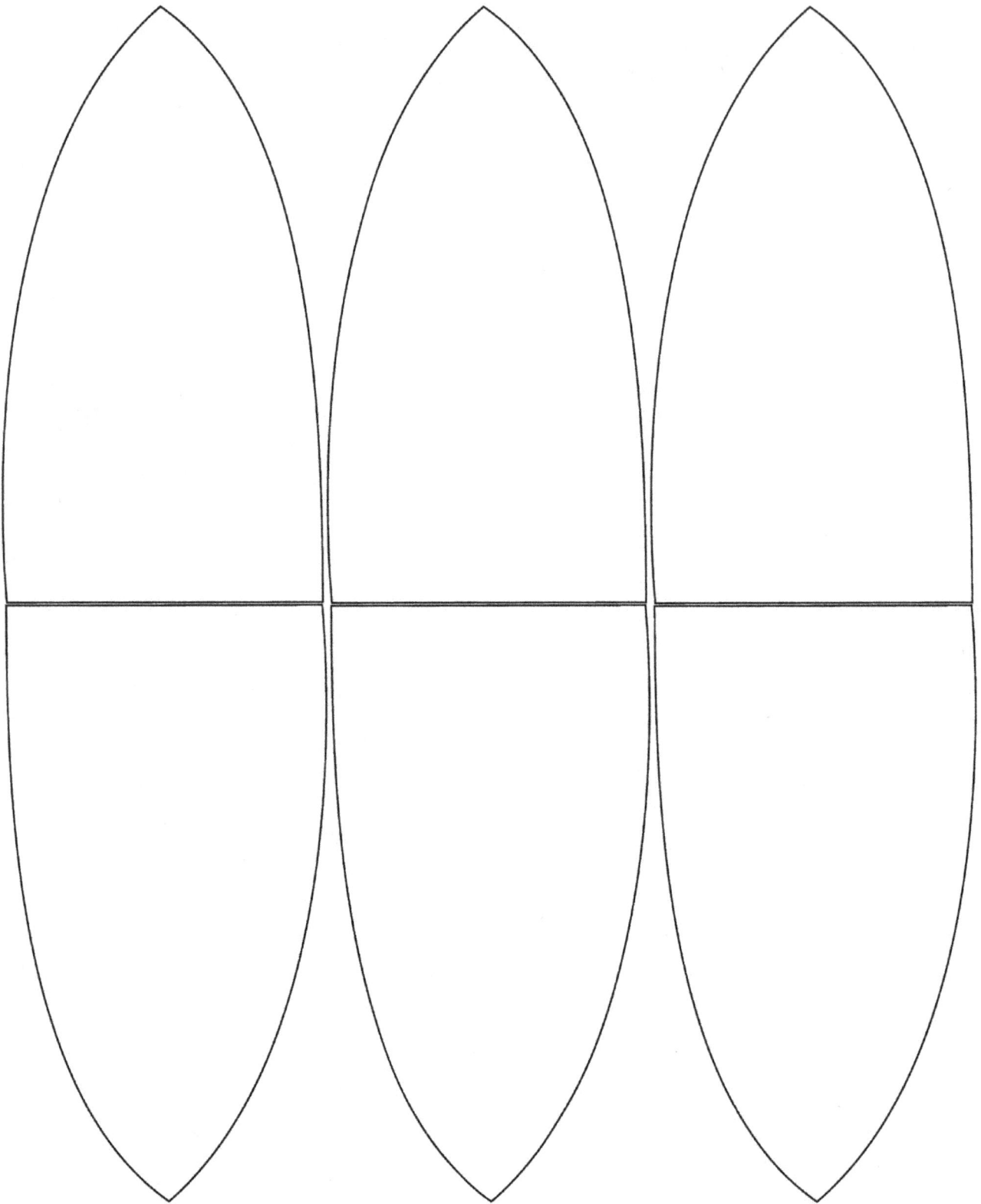

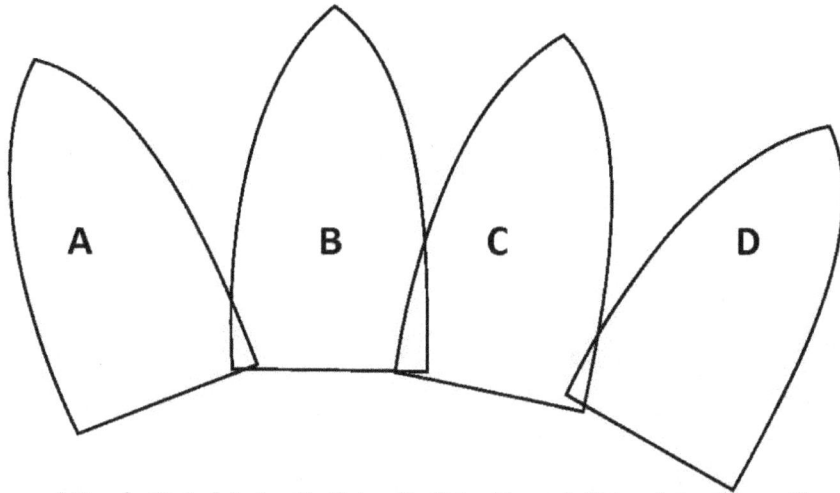

Attach Petal A to B, B to C, C to D and D to A to form the inner ring.

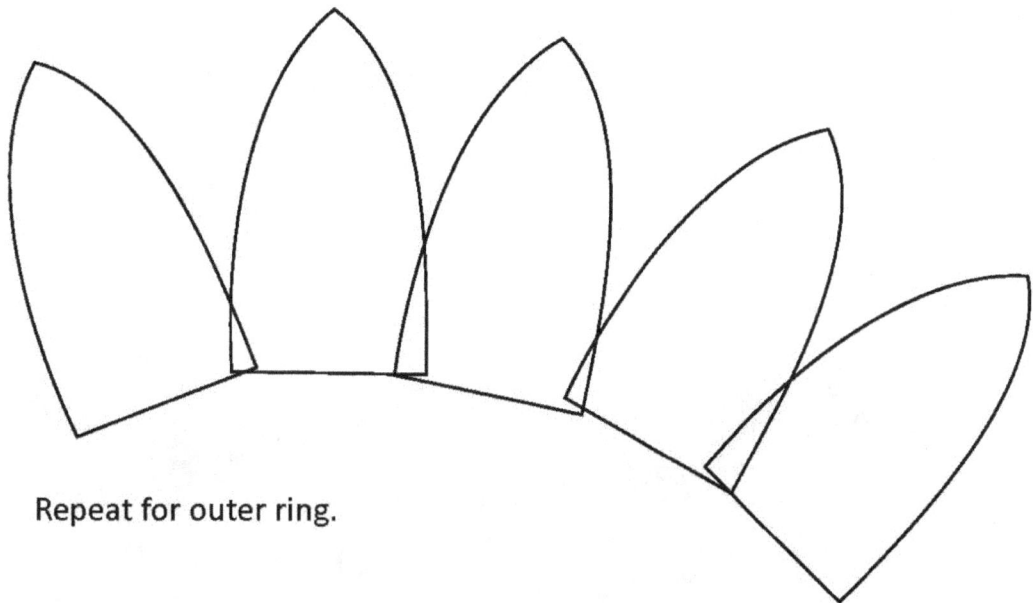

Repeat for outer ring.

Breathing Buddies

Breathing Buddies are special stuffed animals that only come out during Savasana or breath work. They are very shy and will only stay out if it is very quiet.
Have students lie on their backs. When they are quiet, go around the room and place their special buddy on their belly. Speak quietly to keep the class quiet and listening.

Suggested script:
"Very gently, using only your breath, raise your Buddy up and down. Your Breathing Buddy loves this gentle ride and might even fall asleep on your belly so you have to be extra quiet. Feel your Breathing Buddy rise up with your inhale. Feel it lower down with your exhale.
Breathing Buddies travel to all different yoga classes and visit with all different kids. But you might find a stuffed animal or toy at home that works as your Breathing Buddy. They can help us slow down, relax, get less anxious, and maybe help us fall asleep. Try this if you sometimes have trouble sleeping. The Breathing Buddies choose who they want to lie down on. Sometimes they will pick the same person twice and sometimes they want to visit someone new."

After a few minutes, bring the students out of Savasana and have the students hold onto their Buddies as they come up to sitting. They can hold them in their laps.

Closing:
Breathing Buddies have a favorite song, which is the "My Little Light" song. Holding them in our laps, we can sing it with them.

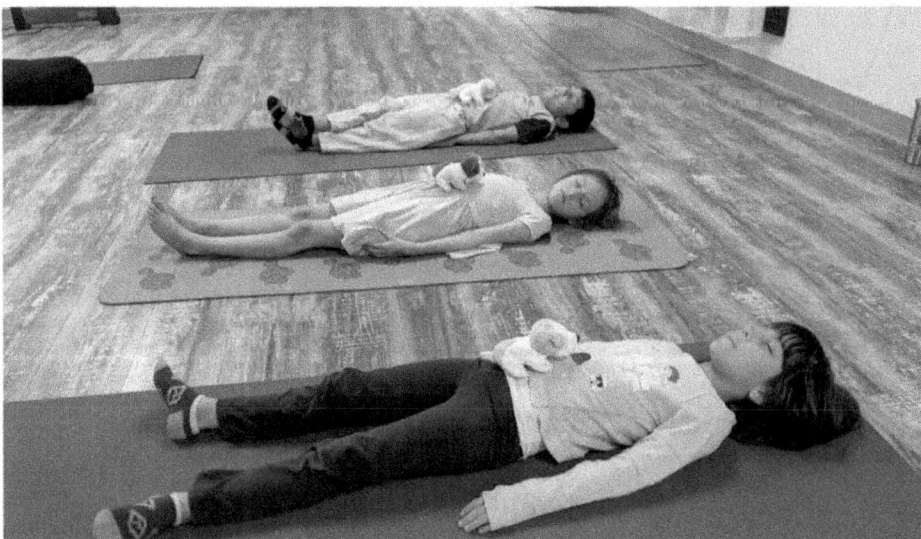

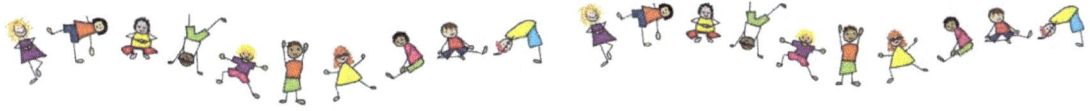

Continue this amazing yoga journey for youth
with the other books in the series:

YOGA FOR KIDS
Lesson Plans for the Teacher

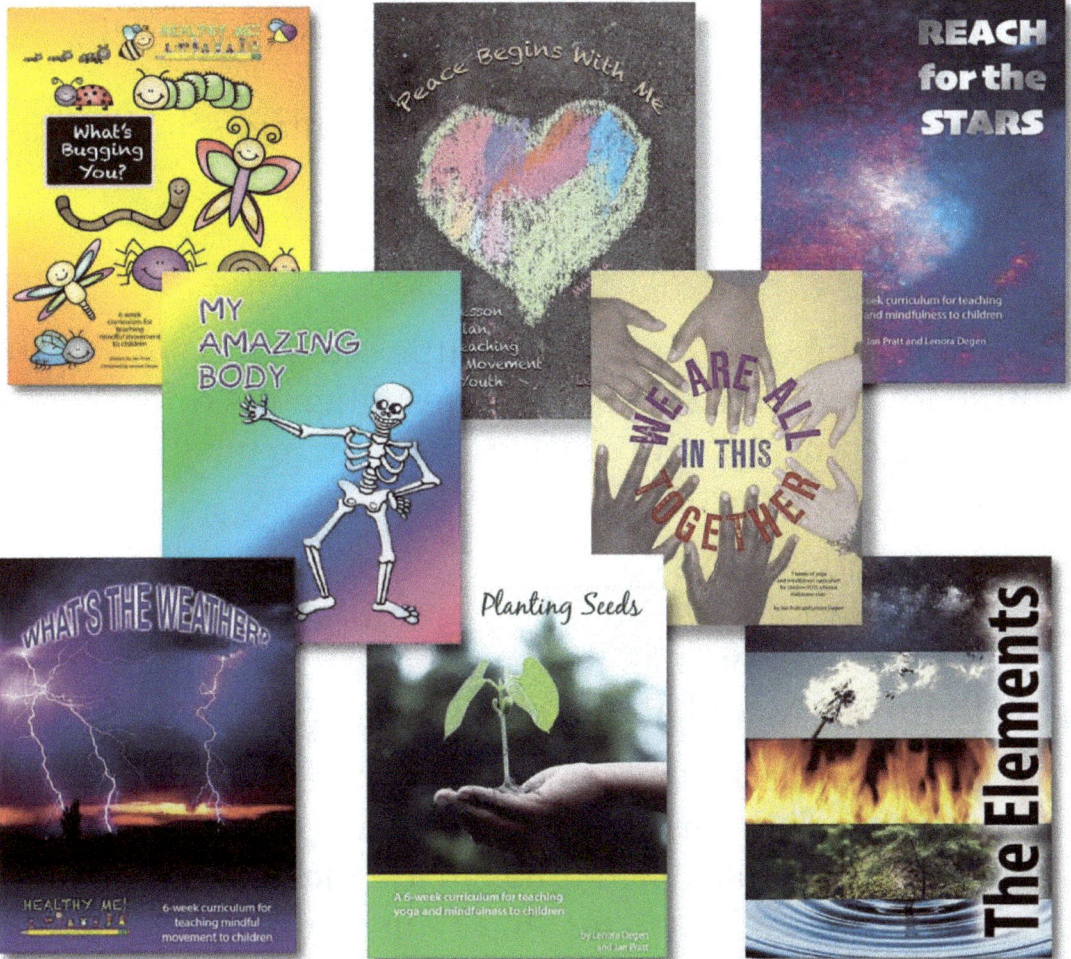

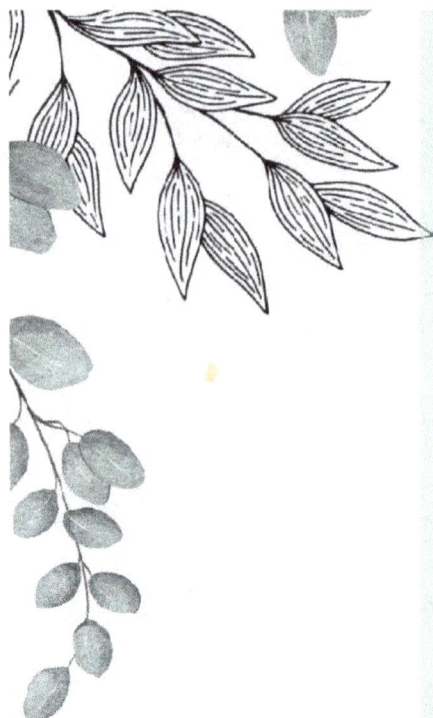

What People Are Saying

"We incorporate yoga into brain breaks in our classroom several times per day.

Yoga is a great way to help create a positive environment, encourage participation, relieve stress, and build self-esteem among my students.

There are so many resources in these curriculum books. Enough to use all school year!"

~ **Ashlee Pape**, elementary school teacher

"Teaching children can be a little scary and a little intimidating. There are times when it's difficult to come up with ideas to keep them busy, engaged, and participating.

Lenora and Janice's curriculum takes all of the worry out of it. It is thoughtful, mindful, engaging–a wide array of all things yoga sprinkled in with fun, easy, and attainable goals.

It includes mindfulness, mantras, games, books, and songs. This curriculum is so easy to follow and never repeats itself. It has made me a better children's yoga instructor, and I am so grateful for the brilliance that Lenora and Janice have put into this and that they share it."

~ **Janine Reed**, yoga teacher

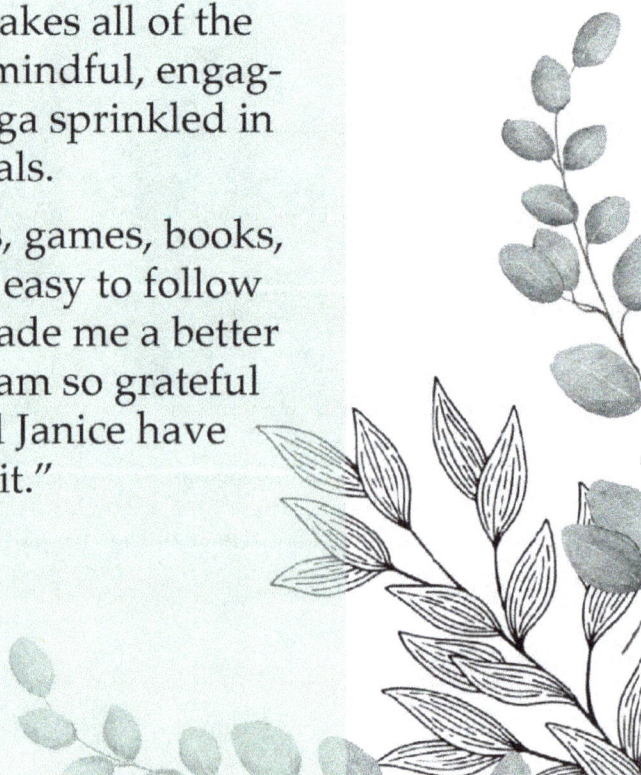

About the Authors

Janice Pratt *(left)*

Ever since I can remember, I have been a reader, often having several books going at the same time. If anyone was my teacher, it has to be the wonderful authors who shared their hearts and souls with me through their stories.

My first story was published in 1999. Today, I work on stories that talk about the amazing power that children have and the mark they can make on the world. I hope to inspire children to feel their truth and know that they can make a difference.

My yoga partner and I created this series to help parents, teachers, and home-school facilitators encourage children of all ages to realize their potential as creative and productive members of our global world.

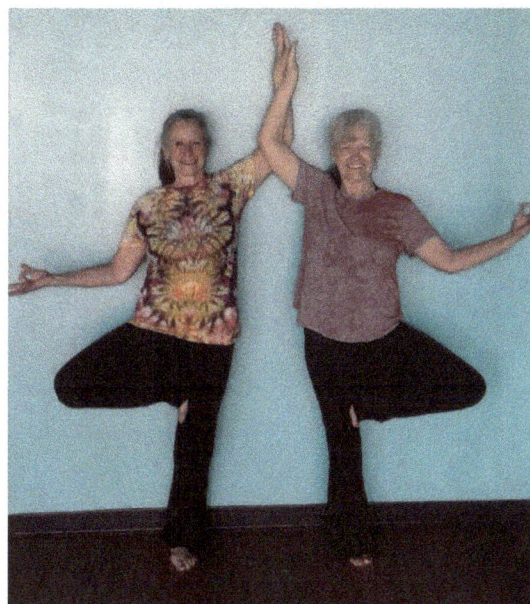

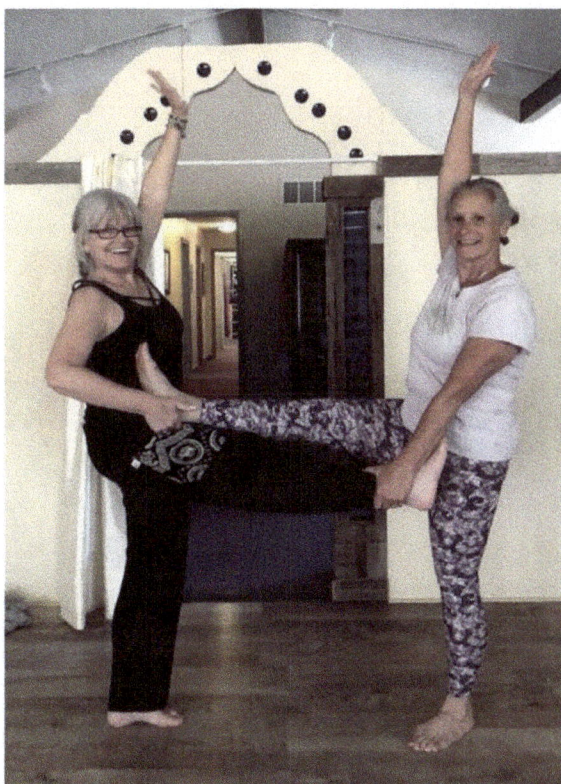

Lenora Degen *(left)*

For the past several years, I have had the amazing privilege of teaching and working with students from 2 - 92 years old! I love bringing the benefits of yoga to people of all ages. I believe there is a form of yoga for everybody on the planet. Working as a creator and graphic designer for the "Yoga for Kids" series, I've had an opportunity to bring two loves of my life together - yoga and graphic design. I hope this curriculum book offers you new and fun ways to share yoga with the young people in your life!

www.ingramcontent.com/pod-product-compliance
Lightning Source LLC
Chambersburg PA
CBHW081201270326
41930CB00014B/3252